Eat Sleep Burn

Dan Garner

CONTENTS

INTRODUCTION

It didn't really begin to unfold until a few years into my coaching practice when I was reviewing yet another new client intake form. You see, before I take on any new clientele I run them through a comprehensive assessment process. At the very end of the questionnaire, I leave the floor open to my new client to voice anything they feel is relevant for the coaching process, I word it exactly like this:

"If there is any other information you feel may be relevant prior to the design of your program, please share it with me below"

The answer to this question, time and time again, revolved around some aspect of a poor night's sleep and reaching out to me for help in this area. Usually along the lines of:

"I have a tough time sleeping well at night, I wake up a few times throughout the night and just don't wake up feeling rested"

"It takes a long time for me to wind down at the end of the day, is there anything you can suggest to help out in this area?"

"I'm exhausted during the day almost everyday. I just don't have the energy I used to" "Getting out of bed and starting my day is impossible without my cup of coffee"

After seeing this continued and repeated pattern, I decided to do a little bit of research behind the prevalence of sleep issues in modern society, and what I came across alarmed me, but didn't surprise me due to the observations I've been making in my practice. To shoot some numbers at you, 67% of all Americans report frequent sleep issues, 43% say that these

sleep issues affect their daily activities, **and between 9-12% of the population is clinically diagnosed with insomnia (Sleep Med. Rev. 2002)**

Beyond this, the Centers for Disease Control (CDC) followed 74,751 adults for their published research in 2011 and they found that 35.3% of people reported less than 7hrs of sleep per night, 38% report unintentionally falling asleep throughout the day, **and 4.7% admitted to falling sleep while driving at least once in the past month** prior to when the survey was conducted (**McKnight-Eily, L.R. 2009**)

To beat you to the calculation, that's 3513 people driving along beside you out there admitting to falling asleep behind the wheel. Keep in mind, these were only the ones who admitted it and was only within a one month timeframe. If that wasn't enough, let me remind you that it was from a survey that only contained 74,751 people. So, if what I'm going to talk about in this book regarding sleep's effect on your fat loss, muscle gain, performance, hormones, immune system, and everything else didn't already want you to read more— you might want to read a little further and help some of your friends just so you don't get hit out there on the road. I know that's not the most positive way to start the book, but it's going to be a bit of a bumpy ride (terrible pun totally intended) over the next few chapters when you realize just how impactful sleep is on our lives.

Naturally, after seeing this trend with my clients and then having it be confirmed by some rock solid data, I wanted to dive further into what type of implications this lack of sleep can have on our lifestyles, health, and ability to reach our goals.

Shouldn't be too bad, right?

It's just sleep, it's not like it's your diet or training or anything.

WRONG

From an everyday life perspective, sleep has been connected to an increase in car crashes, industrial accidents, medical errors, occupational errors; all alongside a reduction in overall life quality and productivity.

From a health perspective, sleep has been connected to chronic disease issues such as high blood pressure, diabetes, depression, obesity, and cancer **(Colten, H. 2006)**

"Alright Dan, I don't have high blood pressure and I don't work in a factory. Can sleep really affect my ability to change my body?"

ABSOLUTELY

Less than 7hrs of sleep per night has been associated to a decrease in athletic performance, increased inflammation, gastrointestinal issues, increased bone loss, poor carb tolerance, increase in catabolic (muscle wasting) hormones, decrease in anabolic (muscle building) hormones, decrease in testosterone, increased food cravings, immune system imbalances, and increased fat gain.

Not to mention, Heymsfield & Gangwisch analyzed NHANES (National Health And Nutrition Examination Survey) data and found that subjects with avg. 5 hr/night sleep had 73% increased likelihood of obesity over those who slept 7-9hr/night.

So, do I have your attention yet? Maybe you don't believe me?

We have a lot of story telling and research to go through my friend…

By unlocking your ability to get a restful night's sleep, you can effectively reverse these issues and launch your health, performance, life quality, and results to the next level. I have done this an untold amount of times in my practice with great success to improve muscle building/fat loss results, in many cases making no changes at all towards an individual's diet or training prescription either.

Sleep length and sleep quality alone are **extremely effective** plateau busters, so if you or someone you know isn't sleep well, this book will provide the next tool they need to keep the results coming in linearly as opposed to hanging around in a plateau.

It is my goal throughout this book to leave no stone unturned and allow you to discover what took me years to realize, dissect, prescribe, and create the now known Sequential Shutdown Method (SSM) to get world class results with my clients and become that "go to" trainer other people seek out when they run into a plateau.

Without further ado, I bring you **EAT, SLEEP, BURN**.

THE MIND-BODY CONNECTION: UNLOCKING YOUR NERVOUS SYSTEM FOR MASSIVE RESULTS

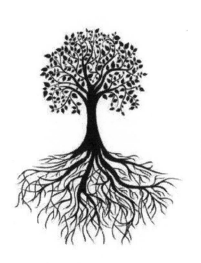 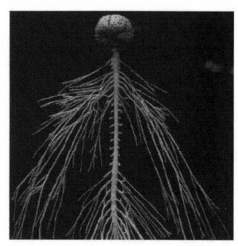

DO THESE LOOK SIMILAR TO YOU?

This is an absolutely brilliant visual comparison that was first taught to me by popular strength coach Elliott Hulse. To the left you have a tree's network system, and to the right we have your brain and nervous system tissue.

What happens if we destroy all the roots of a tree?

It's pretty easy to conceptualize that the tree would die.

That works in reverse too, if we destroy the entire above ground portion of the tree from the grass level up, it's easy to conceptualize that the root system will die. The tree needs both the upper level and lower level in order to sustain its life cycle.

Yet, people so often make the mistake if we parallel that idea to the human body. Think of the upper level as our mind, and the root system as our body. Although they may seem very

different on first thought, the body and mind are not separate entities. They function as one unit just as a tree would. You need both in order to optimize your physiology.

Think the mind doesn't have physical consequences?

Think about somebody who irritates you to your last nerve, yeah that's your heart rate going up. How about that time you were super stressed out?

Did you eat nothing, or did you eat the entire house?

That's the mind impacting your gut in a **very** physical sense.

I think the above picture articulates this idea really well and send the message home. You can see the never ending pathways the brain can take to create a massive impact on the entire body through the "root system" of the nerve tissue, conversely, these highways all lead right back to the brain and can affect our minds in the same manner. This shows you just how connected we really are mind and body, and the actions you decide to take on a daily basis are going to determine whether you have a positive, fat burning, anabolic, and strong connection. Or, a negative, catabolic, fat storing, weak connection.

Who you are is just as physical as what you are. We have to take care of our minds in order to take care of our body, and we have to take care of our body in order to take care of our minds.

For example, **Stults et al in 2014** found that psychological stressors delayed recovery from exercise more than 200% compared to their non-stressed counterparts. The mind affecting the body is a very real, tangible way. Put another way, the above ground part of the tree creating

a negative impact on the underground roots, even though we never touched the roots. If you and your friend are both training together, but you have a more stressful lifestyle, **your friend is going to both recovery faster and be less sore than you.**

Put the energy pathways in reverse now (starting from the roots and going up), elevations or falls in certain hormones levels secreted from areas below the neck can alter brain connectivity, neurotransmission, and even brain structure (**Barth, 2015**); demonstrating the body's ability to dramatically alter the mind.

Menstrual cycles anyone?

How about roid rage?

This is the body affecting the mind. These roads have two lanes, one going up and one going down.

To completely understand performance and getting maximum results, you have to take yourself out of the muscle cell and view the body from both a physiological and psychological standpoint.

Why?

Because they carry equal importance. You can't just have a tree stump, and what good is a dead root system? Like the tree needs its trunk along with its roots, we need our brain working with our body.

Macronutrients, micronutrients, nutrient timing, and energy balance are wildly important; but deep breathing, meditation, having a hobby you love, and feeling fulfilled psychologically and emotionally in your life are just as important.

Until you're mentally ready, you will never be truly physically prepared.

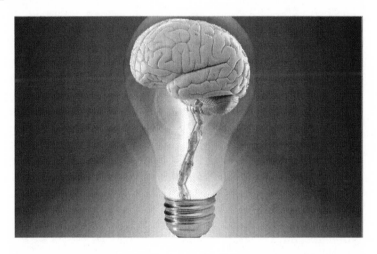

This type of conversation always reminds me to humble brag (not so humble) about a scenario where I was training a young football player in the US, he was 18 years old and a standout in his high school years. Linebacker, but only 188lbs in his senior year. He was able to still play very well and impress people due to his fearlessness and speed, but if you know American football you know that 188lbs linebackers don't last long once you're no longer the big fish in a small pond.

Stuck at 188lbs, his parents called me with him on the phone, told me the situation and I agreed to take him on for the offseason to put some lean mass on the young man. After the assessment, I found out his coaches told him to try to have two Mars bars per day in order to bulk up.

Thank goodness his parents called me. I probably saved this kid a wasted offseason and a pancreas.

He starts up the diet I prescribe him and in the first few weeks go goes from 188lbs to 191lbs. One pound per week (morning weight) gained, I'll take it.

But the next three weeks a whole lot of nothing happened. Getting impatient, his parents and himself asked me for some guidance to keep the momentum going. Before increasing his calories, I sent him over a stress assessment form. Most of the time I won't send 18 year olds this type of assessment, but he was really mature for his age and seemed a little hyper/intense every time I talked to him. I wanted to dig deeper here.

Turns out, he didn't do that well in school and was in summer school for the offseason, which he hated. Beyond that, summer school was a 40mins drive there and back every time he went, which put him on the road 80mins per day, which he also hated. Lastly, he told me he was already nervous about football camps coming up in a couple months where "these big shot older guys" will be watching him and seeing what he's got.

"I see" I said. "Let me write something up for you, you'll have it in your inbox tonight" No, I didn't give him Mars bars.

What I did do was give him a 5-Minute deep breathing routine to follow twice per day. Once upon waking, the next whenever he could fit it in within the afternoon or evening. To be honest I didn't care when the second one came, I just wanted him to get it in. The first one was important though, I wanted him to start the day with a clear mind and allow the deep breathing to calm him down.

Long winded story short?

Two deep breathing sessions per week jumped this kids mass from 191lbs to 193.2lbs that week. Numbers he hasn't seen for a month now, and I didn't even touch his caloric intake.

How does freaky stuff like this happen?

To tell you, we need to talk a little about how the nervous system works.

A NERVOUS SYSTEM OVERVIEW

The nervous system is an incredibly complex organized system consisting of the brain, spinal cord, neurons, neurotransmitters, electrical impulses, nerve fibers, and many other complicated items that won't really do you any good learning.

Although textbooks and other research sources offer fantastic information and is where I learned almost all of what I know about the nervous system, you end up going through a lot of dense, seemingly useless content along the way of picking up what you actually need to know.

I'm going to go ahead and save you the hours of anatomy and physiology memorization that you will never end up using to help you or the people around you and instead, jump right into the meat and potatoes of what you need to know.

First, the nervous system as a whole is composed of two major branches; the central nervous system (CNS) and the peripheral nervous system (PNS). The CNS is composed of the brain and spinal cord, whereas the PNS has two more branches to it that are known as the sensory and motor divisions.

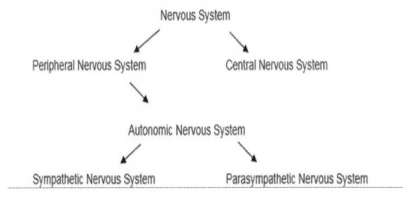

Simplified Breakdown of Nervous System Anatomy

In this document, we are going to focus in on the autonomic nervous system branches known as our sympathetic and parasympathetic systems.

PARASYMPATHETIC DEFINED

Relating to the part of the autonomic nervous system that counterbalances the action of the sympathetic nerves. It consists of nerves arising from the brain and the lower end of the spinal cord and supplying the internal organs, blood vessels, and glands.

SYMPATHETIC DEFINED

Relating to or denoting the part of the autonomic nervous system consisting of nerves arising from ganglia near the middle part of the spinal cord, supplying the internal organs, blood vessels, and glands, and balancing the action of the parasympathetic nerves.

As you can see from the above medical definitions, these two systems completely balance one another and have completely opposing actions. The sympathetic system can be viewed as your "fight or flight" branch, whereas the parasympathetic system can be viewed as your "rest and digest" branch. One is turned on during stressful situations to support immediate survival, the other is turned on during calmer states to support long term health and survival.

PHYSIOLOGICAL NERVOUS SYSTEM CHARACTERISTICS	
Sympathetic State	**Parasympathetic State**
"Fight or flight" system	"Rest and Digest" system
Dilates pupils	Pupils constrict
Increased heart rate	Heart rate normal
Increased respiration	Respiration normal
Increased blood pressure	Blood pressure normal
Blood flow shunted away from the G.I. tract to support limbs	Blood flow within the G.I. tract to support proper digestion and absorption
Systemically *catabolic*	Systemically *anabolic*

(Wilmore, Jack H. Physiology of Sport and Exercise, Human Kinetics. Fourth Edition)

From the above characteristics, you can see that our fight or flight system prepares the body to face a crisis and sustain "alarmism" function during that crisis by producing a massive discharge of chemicals and energy substrates to prepare you for life or death action. A sudden loud noise, life threatening situation, or those last few seconds before the gun fires in a 100m dash are examples I'm sure you can relate to for when this massive discharge occurs.

What's not normally mentioned though is the effects of chronic stress on your body. You see; being stressed out on the road, being in a bad relationship, stressing out about work, **getting consistently poor sleep at night**, among any other kind of "non-life or death" stressor you can think of, still activates sympathetic activity.

Getting chased by a bear? Sympathetic activation. Going on a first date? Sympathetic activation.

The body only knows stress, it doesn't know how silly it is to activate the same survival pathways for a bear attack as it does being nervous on a first date. I think we can all agree a bear in front of us should be a little bit more "cause for concern" then a first date. At least, I certainly hope so!

This is very important to care about because even the low-grade sympathetic activity is still catabolic (breaks down) to your muscle tissue, takes blood away from your G.I. tract which can affect the health of the gut, will increase carbohydrate cravings, increase the risk and severity of depression, reduce thyroid activity which reduces your metabolism, and will actually **lower your testosterone overtime**.

Yes, that's correct. When the body is in a life or death situation, such as being chased down by a hungry lion, it doesn't care about producing testosterone, giving you ab's, or building muscle.

Why?

Because those do not help the life or death situation and will not help you evade the lion. Making testosterone and building muscle can happen later when you're safe and sound, right now, we have to get as far away from this lion as we can and we will only have a chance at doing that if we go sympathetic.

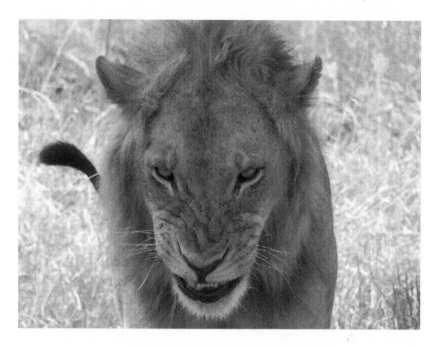

You think you can chill out during this?

But it comes at a physiological cost, you can use the car analogy. If I put the pedal to the metal, I will likely go very fast. But, if I always do that, I will slowly breakdown and deteriorate the car overtime in comparison to if I just drove it like a sane normal person.

The net result of the pedal to the metal lifestyle is hormonal havoc, reproductive dysfunction, muscle loss, and fat gain. Not something we're after, is it?

But what many don't understand is that it doesn't stop there.

With all of these stress hormones and adrenaline being constantly pumped out (due to work stress, relationship stress, overtraining, poor sleeping habits, poor nutrition habits, etc), eventually the adrenal glands begin to slow production of cortisol and adrenaline. This is when chronic fatigue typically begins to set in. You can only put that pedal to the metal for so long until you run out of gas, the body works no different. With chronic stress comes an eventual decrease in stress hormones, or, "gas". (**Duan, H. 2013**)

"But wait, if I'm getting this right Dan, you said that these two branches of the nervous system completely oppose one another. So, if a sympathetic/stressed state lowers testosterone, catabolizes muscle tissue, and decreases our gut health; does a parasympathetic state then increase my testosterone, promote anabolism in my muscle tissue, and improve my gut health?"

Yes, that's exactly right.

Unlocking your nervous system is about three major things:

1.Getting your sleep length and sleep quality to optimal levels

2.Finding balance in your life

3.Using techniques, rituals, and supplements to activate and promote maximal parasympathetic activity

This is where the Sequential Shutdown Method comes in, and how we will be optimizing your physiology to its highest degree throughout the duration of this program.

Since we will be covering your rituals, supplement protocols, and sleep physiology in other chapters, I want to take this time to discuss both life balance and parasympathetic activation techniques with you so you can learn how to switch your anabolic machinery on, and turn your catabolic machinery off. This comes down to a science-based 3-Way chess match between your nervous system, your sleep, and knowing where the switches are.

SWITCHING "OFF" YOUR SNS AND SWITCHING "ON" YOUR PNS

It's not all doom and gloom in this book, there is plenty you can do to unlock and balance your nervous system to promote maximal recovery, quicker results, muscle building, fat loss, and health.

The key here, as stated above, is balance. I'm not going to sit here and tell you "well just don't ever be stressed out"

That wouldn't have worked for Todd, it wouldn't have worked for his wife, and it wouldn't have worked for the agitated football player I previously told you about (who we'll get back to by the way). You can't just tell people to calm down, it doesn't work like that.

Life happens, and life can get in the way of us doing the things we love and reaping the maximal reward of the hard work we are putting into our training and nutrition.

Ever have a hard day at work, or get in a fight with your significant other, and then you go to the gym and you're just not into it? Everything feels like a million pounds, and your mind isn't on the weights?

Yeah, that's because these stress factors take more away from us than just our time, they take our energy, drive, mental capacity, and hormonal homeostasis. (**Ranabir, 2011**)

So since we can't eliminate stress, we must find balance. This means focusing on the PNS side of the equation and hoping for a:

PNS > SNS

Equation by the day's end.

If we can get a little more PNS activity than SNS activity by the end of the day, we're in pretty good shape. But if that's impossible (let's say you have a super stressful job), then at least getting **some PNS activity** by the end of the day is going to be much better than none.

In fact, it's in the already stressed out/intense individuals I see the biggest immediate return on investment from when activating the PNS, even if it is just for 5-10mins a day.

If you're reading this, I'm assuming you're not a yogi on the top of a mountain who has no worries and is in a constant state of Zen (if you are, why did you buy this and how did you find an internet connection?). All of us have some form of stress, whether this be psychological, environmental, emotional, or physical; they all activate similar stress pathways and add to the accumulation of stressors (SNS activation) in our body. (**Schneiderman, N. 2005**)

This means engaging in activities that we love and work for our lifestyle and schedule to switch on the PNS system to promote a state of rest and relaxation is going to help **everybody** reading this take their mind and body to the next level and become a better version of them self.

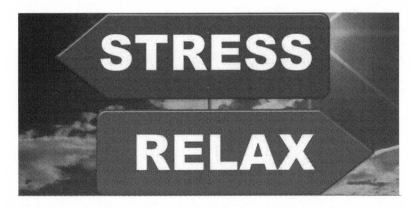

Learning The Techniques To Activate The PNS Outside Of The Gym Puts Your Body In A Restful State And Promotes Maximal Signalling For Physical Change

Some of the most common and demonstrated effective techniques to switch on the PNS within the scientific literature are:

• **Yoga** - Real Yoga though, not all of the modified versions of today that are just basically real workouts. A basic rule to follow is that if it's called anything besides Yoga, don't do it. Yoga pump? Nope. Yoga kick? Hell no. Yoga blast? You've gotta be kidding me. Nobody is going to be activating their PNS while kicking or blasting anything. (**Balaji, 2012**.)

• **Meditation** - My personal favorite, I like to borrow the analogy from a fellow coach named Tommy Hewett using the sport of golf when it comes meditation. Golf can be frustrating at times, but, the moment you smack the ball perfectly and drive that sucker 300yds perfectly down the fairway, or make that perfect putt; these are the moments that keep you coming back for more golf.

That's what meditation is like, in the beginning it can be hard to reach a deep state, but very soon you will smack a dinger down the fairway and realize how powerful and amazing this stuff really is towards your mental state, recovery, and physique progression. Then, just like golf, you will hone your skills overtime and be able to make great shots every time you're up to the tee. Please, no blast-meditation though. I don't even know what that would mean, but I don't put anything past my social media timeline anymore. (**Sharma, 2015**)

• **Massage** - Getting manual treatment is a very effective method in which to activate the PNS and allow you to enter a state of rest and digest. This is technically characterized within the scientific recovery literature as "compassionate touching", and is much less creepy than it sounds. This terminology represents the sports science term for all human contact affecting recovery. This includes other modalities as well such as spa treatments, non-painful tissue work, and even sexual activity. So, whatever floats your boat. (**Sands, W. 2017**)

• **Traditional sauna or Infrared sauna** - Both of these have also been demonstrated to enhance recovery of the body (**Mero, A. 2015**), hence their use in recovery strategies both old school and new school. I also personally lump Epsom salt baths in this scenario as well, even though they do not have anywhere near the scientific data on them that saunas do it is still something I prescribe commonly in my coaching practice.

Why?

They work. That's why. My athletes do recover more efficiently with them, so long as that happens, I'm happy!

Additionally, I am not always the biggest fan of the dehydration and accelerated glycogen depletion that high temperature environments such as saunas can bring (**Galloway, SD. 1997**). But, if you prepare, utilize nutrient timing strategies and hydrate accordingly, they can be used with no issues. Essentially, the body doesn't like anything in extremes. Saunas can be beneficial, but cooking yourself is not. I'd say that's common sense but, you know, there are also people out there that still "Eat for their blood type", so I can't be too careful.

Beyond these strategies, there are some more simple strategies to switch on and activate PNS activity, but they become largely individual at this point due to varying interests and passions.

For example:

• Reading

- Watching the sunset or sunrise

- People watching as you drink your morning coffee

- Zoning out and listening to music

- Lighting candles and watching your favorite movie

- Watching your favorite TV show

- Going for a walk with your dog

(Nobody is parasympathetic around cats, those backstabbers)

Can all be totally viable PNS enhancing activities, so long as you love them and feel rested/ rejuvenated once you do them. It's all about the mind state. The activity you choose doesn't matter. It's the state you achieve. One person could achieve a deep PNS state while relaxing in an Epsom salt bath. While another might just lay in the bath and only think about their money problems. Again, it's the personal state of the individual, not the actual activity itself (provided it's not strenuous of course, I don't care if you **enjoy** Brazilian Jiu-Jitsu. That ain't parasympathetic).

You need to **choose the activities that can help you get a recommended 30 minutes of quiet, restful, worry-free parasympathetic activity each day**. That's the absolute best way to balance and unlock your nervous system to make sure you're always busting through plateaus and not getting stuck in them.

So, remember that football player of mine? That guy who couldn't gain weight and then immediately added a couple pounds to his frame the same week I taught him how to switch on his PNS?

Now you know the **why** behind how this stuff works. A human body can only make progress based on what it can effectively recover

21

from. If you aren't recovering, you also aren't adapting to any stimulus you are trying to create in the gym, and therefore not going to be making any of those gains you are working so hard to get.

When you switch on the PNS, you allow the body the opportunity to "rest and digest" and activate the systems to boost your testosterone, enhance your recover, improve your digestion, become systemically anabolic, and not have to worry about that damn angry lion in your face.

THE SCIENCE OF SLEEP

Sleep is a topic I catch many people off guard with, mainly because they either don't think about it or have underestimated its role in the development of health and having a kick ass body.

When discussions come up involving performance enhancement, the two main topics are training and nutrition, yet sleep is equally as pivotal. If your sleep is off, you're setting yourself up for a lot of problems with your recovery, and if you're creating a lot of problems in recovery you're affecting all aspects of muscle building, fat loss, mental clarity, and performance; among many other things that we're just about to get into.

I like to picture it like a tripod. One leg is training, the second leg is your nutrition, and the third leg is your sleep. If you knock just one of these legs out, the whole stool crashes. Without all three, the foundation collapses.

This is important to care about because almost everybody you meet has a hyper-focus on only the aspects of training and nutrition, but optimal results are without a doubt a complete tripod. If you only attack your training and nutrition, you're leaving **A LOT** on the table.

Put another way, if you bought a stool you wouldn't forget to screw in one of the legs, would you?

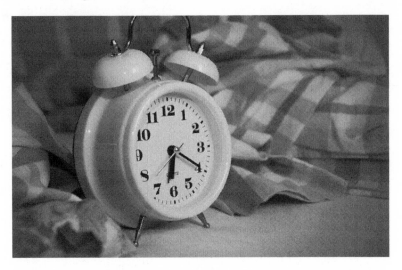

No, because that would be ridiculous.

If there is one thing I want to make very clear here it's that sleep has always been, and always will be your #1 tool for total body and mind recovery. Without sleep it doesn't matter how many calories, supplements, or other fatigue management strategies you use. You will still be tired, you will still be under recovered, you still won't be prepared for optimal exercise, and you will still have disrupted hormonal and immune system function. The SSM feeds on all of these opportunities for enhancement and takes anybody who isn't currently optimizing their sleep quality to the next level in whatever they are trying to accomplish.

I get inquiries for my coaching services all the time, every single day I get e-mails and messages from people wanting to know how I go about training and meal planning for elite results and how I go about the designing process for my world champion athletes.

Then, when it's their turn for programming, they are a little surprised that a sleep questionnaire is its entire own section within my assessment process.

That's right, Dan the training and nutrition man sends out a questionnaire exclusively dedicated to asking specific questions about your sleeping habits before I ever start putting pen to paper on your plan.

And you know what?

If they don't fill it out I won't do their programming, it's a part of the assessment process for a reason. You try coaching somebody to sit on a stool with only two legs. Go ahead, try it.

We both (coach and client) need to know the state of your sleep length and sleep quality because having a discussion about maximizing your life while leaving sleep out of the conversation would be an incomplete program and an incomplete assessment that would lead to incomplete results.

Why would I leave a whole leg of the tripod out before I started putting pen to paper on your programming?

I never would.

I've had many cases in my career where sleep alone was the reason why somebody was plateauing in their muscle gain or fat loss. It had nothing to do with the gym and it had nothing to do with their diet. It had **everything** to do with what they do between the hours of 10pm and 6am.

Here's the thing, sleep is supposed to be natural, not difficult. If you're having big troubles falling asleep and staying asleep at night, this is an obvious red flag.

Why is the body not properly making the chemicals it needs for sedation and sleep? This is supposed to happen without you even thinking about it, like an automatic internal clock.

This is what this program is all about:

• Answering those questions of dysfunction

• Articulating the consequences of sleep dysfunction on different tissues and systems in the body

• And finally providing you with the information and protocols necessary to maximize your results and crush your goals.

Since knowledge is power, let's get into it.

SLEEP'S EFFECT ON HORMONES, THE BRAIN, AND YOUR MUSCLE DEVELOPMENT

Most all systems in the body become anabolic during sleep. This includes your bone, immune, nervous system, muscle tissue, and endocrine systems. During the night, the bones are building up and remodeling, muscle tissue is being added to the body, and various systems are producing hormones such as growth hormone (GH) and testosterone at their peak levels (**Sharma, 2010**).

Very important note here: The gym is where you create **only a stimulus** for muscle growth, where the process of lifting weights sends the signal to the body "Holy crap! That was heavy! We better adapt by building some muscle and getting stronger!"

But, this is just a stimulus. A signal for growth, if you will.

The actual tissue growth occurs only during a quality recovery, which demands a good night's sleep. Train to stimulate, sleep and recover to adapt. Stimulation alone is just a stimulus, that's why training is only one leg of the stool, while both nutrition and sleep are needed to ensure you actually recover and adapt from that stimulus.

The accumulation of sleep research has shown comparing 5 hours of sleep to 8 hours of sleep that the groups who consistently had less sleep have higher concentrations of catabolic

(muscle breakdown) hormones such as cortisol, and also had lower concentrations of anabolic (muscle building) hormones such as testosterone and IGF-1. In fact, one study out of the University of Chicago demonstrated a 14% decrease in testosterone in healthy men once they decreased their sleep from 9hrs a night to 5hrs per night (**Leproult, 2011**).

Additionally, neurotransmitter pools in the brain are being restocked and contributing to all sorts of different metabolic benefits to our daily lives. But most of which being relevant to you include increased motivation, drive, focus, speed of thought, speed of muscle contraction, learning, memory, attention span, vasodilation, and reduced time to fatigue. All contributing not only to physical performance but also mental performance, that's powerful stuff right there.

It's important to care about mental performance as well because the more in the zone you can be, the better you can execute your technical lifts and train the way you need to train in order to get maximum results in the shortest time frame.

If we have continuous stressors coming in, such as mental (Ex. an exam, or our job), emotional (Ex. relationship problems with your significant other, family, or with yourself), or physical events (Ex. training, manual labor work) in our lives; the combination of stress damage and poor sleep can wreak havoc on how these neurotransmitters operate and what our mental state is going to be like on a day to day basis (**Kinner, VL. 2006, Watson, J. 2010**) Not to mention it is enormously catabolic to your hard earned muscle tissue (**Gore, 1993**).

The performance benefits are somewhat common sense. Yes of course there are many cellular intricacies that go into the "why" behind that but just looking at it bluntly, if you're one of these people who is chronically tired, your performance is clearly going to suffer. There's no way around that and you probably didn't need me to tell you that.

But from a body composition standpoint it isn't so common sense.

When most of you think of making changes to your body or physical performance, you're going look to training, nutrition, and probably some supplements. Which don't get me wrong, those three things are a totally great place to start. But when viewing the total potential for change from a whole picture point of view, leaving out sleep is leaving out a big chunk of what you could be accomplishing.

Within the muscle building and fat loss vein, sleep's effect on the body's Respiratory Exchange Ratio (RER) is one of its biggest noticeable and dramatic effects. RER is a way in which to measure the primary source of your body's fuel that it is going to use for its energy needs.

If you have a low measured RER (they measure this stuff in labs, but that's not important to get the overall idea) you are burning a greater proportion of fat per day to meet your energy needs.

Not bad, right?

But if you have a high measured RER, you guessed it, your body is burning a greater proportion of lean tissue per day to meet in order to meet its basal energy needs.

Keeping in mind the above difference between low and high RER rates, most of us are all also familiar with Basal Metabolic Rates (BMR). For those of you who are not familiar, a BMR value is the number of calories at which you burn per day just to sustain normal bodily function. This is the rate of energy the body uses while at rest to keep vital functions going, such as breathing, having your organs work without you needing to think about it, and keeping your temperature stable. This can vary quite a bit between individuals based primarily on size. For example, a 300lbs strongman competitor is going to have a higher BMR to keep his body functioning on a day to day basis than a 90lbs couch potato. Bigger machines need more fuel.

Where RER values come back into play is that they determine how much of this base daily calorie burn is coming from either fatty tissue, or lean tissue (muscle and glycogen stores). If you're reading this program, it is very likely that you want to have a respectable lean muscle tissue to fat tissue ratio so that you have a lean, aesthetic physique. By default of this goal, optimizing RER is something of significant importance here because you want to be burning fat**, NOT YOUR HARD EARNED MUSCLE.**

How sleep ties into this is research has shown that **low levels of sleep (5.5hrs nightly) significantly raises your RER**. Meaning, if you are consistently getting poor sleeps you are shifting the majority of your daily calorie burn to lean tissue as opposed to fatty tissue. Ideally, we would have a low RER value to optimize fat burning while keeping your lean muscle mass.

That's how you sculpt a physique, not matter what your end goal is. Want to look like a bodybuilder?

How about like a bikini model?

What if you just want to look athletic?

Or, if you're conservative and just want to be a little healthier and have some more energy? All of those things involve RER, and ultimately, sleep.

Here's some more bad news for the poor sleepers, if I haven't brought enough of that already throughout this book.

A decreased sleep level raises your RER value without affecting your basal metabolic rate. Meaning, if your daily calorie burn average is 2500 calories, it is going to stay that way with or without a bad sleep. So, if you get a bad sleep and your RER raises, your metabolism won't lower to offer up some damage control. You will just lose that much more lean tissue. A high metabolism combined with a high RER means a whole lot of unnecessary muscle loss due to a factor that is totally independent of nutrition and training.

To put things into perspective and give some examples. Let's say you have an average calorie burn of 2500 calories per day. If you have a low RER value, 2000 of that could be coming from fat and only 500 from lean tissue. Whereas if you have a high RER value, 1250 could be coming from fat at 1250 from lean muscle tissue. Not a good trade off if optimizing your performance potential and body composition are in your sights.

Why should we actually care about this?

I can quickly answer this question with a couple other questions.

If you're trying to lose weight, do you want to lose 50% body fat and 50% lean muscle tissue? Or would you rather lose a lot more body fat and not any lean muscle tissue?

If your priorities are straight and you're looking to keep and/or build as much lean muscle mass as you can while decreasing your body fat percentage, the latter is the obvious option and getting a great night's sleep is an effective tool in your arsenal.

This also works in the other direction.

If you're trying to **gain** weight and lean muscle mass but you sleep poorly on a regular basis, you're going to be spinning your tires in the mud. Going nowhere **fast**. You will simultaneously have a higher amount of catabolic hormones (cortisol), a lower amount of anabolic hormones (testosterone, IGF-1), lower neurotransmitter pools, and a high RER value. Good luck with that!

If laying out the theory wasn't enough, this RER work was demonstrated in some research done at the University of Chicago where 10 overweight adults followed a weight loss diet for two weeks. One group slept for 8.5hrs per night, while the other group was restricted to only sleep for 5.5hrs per night. The results were striking.

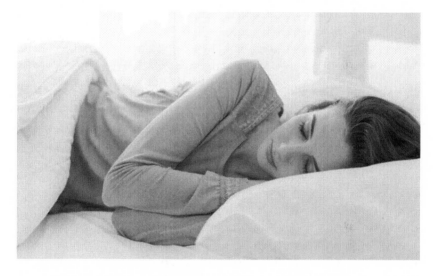

The 5.5hrs of sleep per night group lost 55% less fat and 60% more muscle than the 8.5hrs of sleep per night group. Beyond this, the 5.5hrs group also reported greater

cravings than the 8.5hrs group, lending susceptibility to the idea that not only were they burning muscle instead of fat, but they were also more likely to cheat on their diet that day as well (**Nedeltcheva, A. 2011**)

SLEEP AND THE IMMUNE SYSTEM

A very important factor to consider as well here is sleep's effect on your immune system function. One thing that I was taught early on from a coach is that your ability to put on muscle mass is largely predicated on how well-functioning your immune system is.

Always getting sick?

It's likely your immune system is not functioning properly for some underlying reason, and when the immune system isn't functioning normally you cannot expect to respond and recover from exercise optimally as it is your immune system that is largely involved in both the signalling for progress and the actual recovery-adaptation phase as well. (**Brunelli, S. 2008**)

Sleep directly affects the immune system in the exact way you think it does: Good sleeps = A-OK immune function

Bad sleeps = Not so good immune function

We need the immune system firing on all cylinders because it is the immune system that is helping you recover from exercise and from all the other activities/sports you do. Any intense physical activity is a temporary knock at the immune system and the immune system has to recover from the exercise bout and still try to protect you from illness while it's at it. The more intense physical bouts you partake in, the more hits you're placing on your immune system (**Pedersen, BK. 1998).**

A case study example on immune function from exercise can be brought in from fighters getting ready for the big fight. It happens so often that fighters go into a fight ill, or become ill 1 or 2 weeks out from a fight. This is because they have been training so hard during training camp that their immune system could only keep up for so long. A good diet, proper fatigue

management and a good night's sleep are the best tools to fight this immune depression so you can keep training harder and remain free of illness.

Now, we know we need the immune system to recover you from training and from your other activities/sports you partake in, but we also need it to make you get results faster than those around you.

How does my immune system allow me to get faster results?

Well, the more often you get sick the less you can train. This will directly affect your skill development in the technical lifts that can take years to master. Additionally, the more often you get sick the more workouts you are going to miss, or if you attend these "sick workouts" you will have a lower level of potential physical output which overtime will directly affect the results you will receive in a giving time frame.

Think about it, if you are somebody who gets a cold or gets sick once a month or once every two months, this adds up to a lot of bad or totally missed sessions by the year's end when you could have otherwise been training hard and getting results.

The research really backs up these immune connections as well, Carnegie Mellon University researchers assessed the quality and quantity of people's sleep at the time the cold virus was introduced and found that those who were sleeping inefficiently and getting less than seven hours of sleep were three times more likely to get sick compared to people who got eight or more hours of sleep. Even 15 additional minutes of sleep helped improve immunity. A lack of sleep suppresses the body's immune system, making it easier to get sick (**Carnegie Mellon University**)

On a even more extreme level, if you're sleep deprived when you get a flu shot, the efficacy of that shot is reduced. A University of Chicago study of sleep deprivation at the time of flu vaccination showed a 50 percent lower vaccine effectiveness for sleep-deprived people. The

effect wasn't just immediate either, the deficit in immunization effectiveness lasted up to 30 days afterwards. (**Puro, V. 2002**)

This connection between sleep and immunity plays a huge role and effect on your physiology and is something you need to keep in the forefront of your thought process towards recovery and development philosophies moving forward.

SLEEP AND FAT GAIN

Sleep and the fat mass equation can be sometimes be difficult to initially conceptualize given that you are just lying in bed for a period of time, what could that possibly do for fat loss right?

We have to move to burn, don't we?

Turns out it's a little more complicated than that.

It's first important to point out that your body still burns fat while you sleep (Ex. The average 160lb person will burn about 70kcal per hour of sleep, mostly from body fat) because you are in a fasted state and still alive. This whole "living" thing does burn calories you know. Beyond this, growth hormone is heavily stimulated during hours of rest which perpetuates the fat loss efforts (**Sasson, JF. 1969, Takahashi, Y. 1968**)

Knowing this, it's a little bit easier to digest and accept the reality that sleep plays a role in the amount of body fat we carry on our bodies (you know, if the RER wasn't already enough).

Research is also unwinding a vicious cycle between fat gain and sleep, going in both directions. Poor sleep quality increases levels of body fat, while increased levels of body fat lead to further decreased sleep quality. Definitely not a cycle you want to be in. This is a result of the already discussed factors, but also some further hormonal disruption affecting our appetite signalling within the brain.

In one study, subjects who averaged 4hrs of sleep a night or less (**<u>Spiegel, K. 2004</u>**):

• Decreased their leptin hormone concentration by 18% (a hormone which gives feelings of fullness and is a major regulator of a healthy metabolism in the body)

• Increased their levels of the hormone ghrelin by 28% (a hormone which increases hunger and cravings)

• Increased their level of perceived cravings/hunger by 24% (especially towards sweets, salty snack, and high starch foods)

These percentages are huge and all create meaningful differences within our metabolism that can directly impact our health and make us be much more likely to not be able to resist temptations that day.

One temptation isn't bad at all, but, if you add those small battles up over an extended period of time, they can result in the oh so familiar:

"Why doesn't my shirt fit anymore? How did I get this far?"

This type of sleep deprivation-induced overeating effect was very powerfully demonstrated in a study on women that found just four days of sleeping only 6hrs per night increased their voluntary calorie intake by 20% (**Bosy-Westphal, A. 2008**). That is a very fast, and very impactful effect on appetite signalling. To transfer those results into real world terms, let's say you are currently eating 5 equal meals per day (20% of your calories in each meal). Well, just due to sleep deprivation alone you are now bumping your intake up to 6 equal meals per day (20% in each meal, now equalling 120% of your original intake which will undoubtedly lead to weight gain).

In another study with more than a 1000 volunteers involved, they found that those who averaged 5hrs of sleep a night or less had also decreased their leptin and increased their ghrelin. But unique to this research, this population also increased their Body Mass Index (BMI) 3.6% (**Mignot et al. Stanford School of Med. Dec. 2004**)

Now 3.6% may not sound like a lot to many of you when it comes to weight gain, but these results were found irrespective of the subjects diet or exercise habits. Meaning, **just sleep alone showed an increase in BMI no matter how they ate or trained.**

If that wasn't already enough connections between sleep and fat gain, **decreased sleep can also disrupt blood sugar regulation.** One study showing that cutting back sleep to 4hrs a night demonstrated a 40% longer rate to regular blood sugar after a high carb meal, alongside a decreased insulin response of 30% (**Spiegel, K. 1999**).

What does that mean for you?

Elevated blood sugars causing inflammation in your system, likely "sugar crashes" after carb meals, and less of a muscle building anabolic response due to the 30% reduction in the muscle building anabolic hormone insulin. Not to mention, multiple studies have now pointed towards sleep loss presenting blood sugar dysregulation issues that rival Type ll Diabetics, which creates an internal environment where you are much more susceptible to increase the rate at which your body stores carbohydrates as fat (**Jitomir, J. 2009**).

These numbers on blood sugar dysregulation are both relatively and absolutely huge, given the fact that carbohydrate intake and timing are a major part of proper meal planning for the

population interested in making significant body composition changes, it makes a big difference to you directly.

If you're somebody who wants fast and killer results and you're hell bound on making the best progress possible with this program, then carbs should be in your meal plan in the right doses and at the right times. But even if your meal plan is bang on point (and your training for that matter), poor sleep can disrupt how well you manage these carbohydrates in your bloodstream which can lead to unnecessary inflammation alongside a host of other issues.

The effect of sleep is dramatic, in one last study I am going to cover within this category, we saw women build muscle and lose fat over the course of a year by doing absolutely nothing except improving sleep quality (**Amstrup, AK. 2016**). Yes, you read that correctly.

No training.

No diet.

No steroids.

Improving the test subjects sleep quality (via melatonin) alone allowed them to achieve both fat loss and muscle gain without any other factors involved across the year, and accomplish this without any undesirable/unsafe either.

SLEEP AND PERFORMANCE

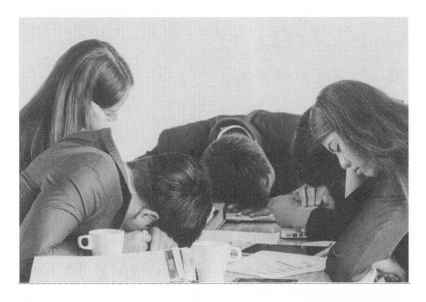

Although your immediate gut reaction may tell you that strength and speed dramatically declines when you have a bad sleep, the research surprisingly tells us otherwise. What we have seen throughout several studies is the emerging idea that sleep largely decreases the mind's ability to **want** to exercise, as well as the minds over-exaggerated **perception** of how difficult your physical activity is. But, the actual true physical potential of muscle tissue is still intact if the dire situation presents itself. Essentially, you still have your force production ability, you will just be faced with the double inertia layers of:

a)Starting exercise

b)Continuing exercise after the going gets tough

To run through a few examples, a study done within the Imam Khomeini International University demonstrated that a single night of sleep deprivation did not affect anaerobic power output in the participants, but it did reduce their reaction time to a statistically significant degree (**Taheri, 2012**). To put it short, you're strong but slow. You're going full Neanderthal on everybody.

Another study within this realm had participants undergo 60hrs of sleep deprivation (Nearly 3 days!) and perform forearm and leg exercises. What was found at the end of the research was that the sleep deprived group performed just as well as their non-sleep deprived counterparts who slept 7hrs per night (**Symons, J. 1988**).

Although, continuing research from this program demonstrated that sleep deprivation results in a faster time to fatigue and a greater perceived exertion per unit of activity performed (**VanHelder, T. 1989**). Put another way, you're tired from not sleeping, so your body wants to quit sooner. It's sending you signals to quit sooner even though your muscles are technically capable of completing the work. You can compare this to the times you have walked up to the bar with a weight you have handled many times before without issues, but for some reason today it feels like it has been loaded with million pounds.

These are the times you pick up a weight you have done before and think: "What the hell is wrong with me today?"

Self perceived exertion is incredibly high, but your true physical ability can handle the weight.

What we can gather from the results we have seen in the literature towards performance and sleep is that you probably don't have to skip your workout today if you slept poorly last night, your muscular potential will still be able to execute.

But, it will feel harder and you will likely have a quicker time to fatigue where you think "Alright, I'm leaving the gym". I can back this up with personal anecdote from myself and from my clients as well. If I sleep poorly once, I don't normally have a bad training session the next day. I will typically only have a bad training session if I have slept poorly 2 or more nights in a row. Then the sleep deprivation truly catches up to me and begins to dramatically alter my self-perceived exertion through every movement. Three nights of bad sleep in a row for me makes me have to listen to a 1-Hour Anthony Robbins speech to even meal prep, let alone squat.

Long story short, you don't need to skip your gym workout if you sleep bad once, your performance will still be there waiting for you. You just need to psyche up and get past the initial inertia.

But, if you're an athlete who is about to compete you might have a greater chance of losing the competition from only one night's bad sleep. There is much wisdom in the old school coaches "Lights out at 10pm tonight!" speech the day before the big game. This is because poor sleep quality even in a single night will alter your speed of thinking and reaction time. Neanderthals don't win championships.

SLEEP QUALITY STRATEGIES

Now that we have gone over some important and relevant sleep research, consequences, and factors as to why you should care about sleep and what sleep can do for your muscle

building, fat loss, mind state, and performance; it's important to also talk about some strategies in which you can use today to start taking advantage of this. Information without action is just information. It can make you sound smart at parties, but you're no more useful than you were without it.

Transforming information into action is what brings everything to a practical and beneficial level. The Sequential Shutdown Method does this in the most complete way possible, but we'll tie that all together in the end. For now, let's just talk about some immediately applicable "one-off" strategies that you **need to know** in order to make sure you're taking advantage of everything we have discussed thus far within this book.

Strategies to improve your quality of sleep include:

• Adequate hydration and timing of hydration throughout the day

• Completely pitch black room to sleep in

• Unplug all electrical equipment in your room

• Do not have your phone on or use it as an alarm

• Getting up and going to bed at the same time every day and night

• Deal with your pre-bed anxiety

• Try to calm down at night time. Nobody ever went to bed relaxed and ready to properly sleep just after watching UFC or action movies. Not going to happen. Reading leisurely (not researching or planning) is a great way to calm down and prime your body for rest.

• No TV or cellphone within 2hrs of bedtime

• Not having every light on in the house after 6pm. The body responds to light as if it is day time and this can delay the proper production of melatonin, a sleep hormone that is necessary for you to be able to fall asleep and stay asleep

These strategies will take you a **long** way in your pursuit of sleeping better. In many cases, this is all that people need in order to change their lives. We'll dive deeper into these and other strategies as well for those of you who want more and want to take every last bit of advantage here within the chapter covering The 10 Rules to Getting the Perfect Night's Sleep.

One last thing that is important to note here within this Science of Sleep chapter is that there is no optimal amount of sleep you should be trying to target, there is only an optimal amount of sleep for **YOU**. Some people only need 7hrs, some people need up to 10hrs per night. The idea is to get enough to where you feel your best. If you can function throughout the day at a

high level without massive doses of caffeine, then you're probably doing pretty good. But if you are chronically under rested, aren't getting results as fast as you think you should be, and feel like a dead person without your pre-workout energy drink, then sleep should be your #1 priority before anything else.

A good rule I like to use when it comes to determining your personal sleep length requirement is that you should never wake up with an alarm. This gets people out of the idea of thinking they must sleep 8 or 9hrs. If 7hrs is good for you and you're not being interrupted by an alarm doing this, by all means go for it. Don't force yourself to sleep in.

I've had athletes on all ends of the spectrum here, some people habitually sleeping only 6hrs per night with no issues, while others need their 10hrs or else their mind and performance suffers. Although we have a large amount of research on varying levels of sleep length and its impact on our physiology, I still consider this component of human performance largely subject to individual variance. We carry many similarities, but we are different.

Some factors directly affect our sleep length, for example, teenagers need roughly 10hrs per night to support their growth and development, whereas the average adults' need drops off much lower within the 7-8hrs per night range. Physical activity level can also increase or

decrease sleep needs, but these factors don't matter in the end if you wake up without an alarm because it will all sort itself out. Your "inner-intelligence" will know how much sleep you need when you go to bed and wake up. Alarms, partying, stimulants, and various other things muck this up and make it hard to determine where somebody's true sleep length requirements lie.

It should also be noted here that "more is better" isn't true. You will not be gaining any advantage sleeping 12hrs a night if your body doesn't need to for adequate recovery. Simply waking up without an alarm is ensuring you are doing it right. There is no trophy for the person who can sleep the longest. Not to mention, data exists as well that sleep too long can disrupt blood sugar regulation in similar mechanisms as sleeping too little can (**Cappuccio, FP. 2010**). When it comes to almost all things in human performance, **more is not better.**

Additionally, research has shown that proper supplementation can have an excellent benefit on both your sleep length and sleep quality, but it's important you use the correct protocols for your current issues, goals, and situation. The Sequential Shutdown Method covers all of this

and your exact needs are going to be met and discussed in a bit. For now, hang tight as there is always a foundation that needs to be placed first before we get into protocol talk.

What are the main takeaways?

It is important to understand that sleep plays a large role in:

• Circadian rhythm (sleep/wake cycles)

• Muscle cell repair and growth

• Fat loss potential

• Fatigue management in preventing overtraining

• Hunger and cravings

• Immune system function

• Endocrine system function

• Blood sugar regulation

• Anabolic hormone production

• Catabolic hormone production

• Respiratory Exchange Ratio (RER)

• Neurotransmitter pools in the brain

My goal with this chapter was to heavily support the importance of sleep and educate you with concrete scientific evidence so that you understand fully and completely that human performance is not a belief system or an idea. That's not how I treat my clients and it's not how I'm writing this book.

Human performance is built from both experience and rock-solid evidence, if we don't have the proper literature behind what we are recommending then we don't have a solid ground in which to make educated decisions from. The science has to be there or else we are just guessing, and guessing doesn't get anybody results. One thing that I want you to take from this chapter is that the recommendations you follow should always have a basis of sound research behind them.

The internet did an amazing thing in the past 10 years for the fitness industry because it gave everybody a voice in the game, but the internet also did a terrible thing for the fitness industry in the past 10 years because it gave everybody a voice in the game. This same thing is a double- edged sword because for everybody well-researched and balanced opinion you read online, there are about 15 more emotionally bias and scienceless ones that are posted at the same time.

Training, nutrition, and human performance are not about opinions. We aren't talking about who is going to win the Stanley Cup this year, we are talking about objective physiology with objective data behind it. Your success in how well you navigate the new world of online health and fitness depends largely on your ability to approach new concepts with a critical-mindset and ask for references or further information when claims are made.

Ultimately, the research supports that the results you get with your physique and the results that you get with your performance depend largely upon on how well, or how poorly you sleep. Do not forget that this is all about balancing the tripod and making sure all three legs of the stool are treated with the same respect.

THE 10 RULES OF GETTING THE PERFECT NIGHT'S SLEEP

Sleep is a topic I have caught many people off guard with. Most all people think of supplements, training, and nutrition when it comes to their health, normally in that order too. But as you have learned throughout this book in extensive detail, sleep is equally as pivotal.

Sleep provides the non-negotiable foundation of your recovery, hormone production, appetite regulation, blood sugar stability, stress hormone release, body fat to muscle gain ratio, mood, among many other vital components towards long term health and having a kick ass physique. So without further ado, let's get into the 10 crucially important rules you must follow in order to enhance both your sleep length and sleep quality.

#1: OPTIMAL HYDRATION STRATEGIES AND HYDRATION TIMING

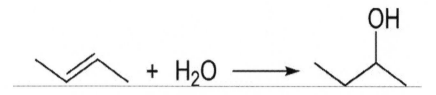

Water Molecule Structure

I know hydration may not be the first thing to come to mind for you when it comes to optimizing sleep length and sleep quality. But let me ask you two things:

1.How much water do you drink per day?

2.Do you get up at night to go to the bathroom?

If you can't answer #1 and you're thinking you drink probably less than you require, you've got a stress hormone problem. What we know from research is that even slight levels of dehydration cause elevations in bodily stress hormones, of particular significance here is the hormone cortisol (**Maresh, CM. 2006**). Not only is this hormone catabolic (muscle wasting), but it promotes wakefulness. So not only can dehydration play into muscle loss (this shouldn't come as a surprise, especially given that muscle is literally 75% water) but it can also directly affect the chemical and hormone signalling process that is supposed to be occurring later in the day to optimize sleep quality.

If the answer to #2 is yes, then you are disrupting your deep wave sleep cycles and negatively affecting your sleep quality. We have seen in some excellent research in this area dating all the way back in 2002, to directly quote the findings:

"Sleep is an essential biological process that is both highly regulated and very complex. Disturbances to the normal pattern of sleep lead to daytime symptoms (fatigue, sleepiness, mood changes), and increased morbidity and mortality. Nocturia, a very common condition that has many causes, results in sleep fragmentation and a reduced quality of life. Recent evidence suggests that in professionally active individuals, nocturia can lead to activity impairment and reduced productivity at work." (**Jennum, P. 2002)**

Aim for ½ your bodyweight in ounces of water per day as a standard baseline. For example, if you are 200lbs you would have a minimum daily intake of 100oz water daily. Beyond this, it is ideal you complete the large majority of this intake with 2hrs still left in your day. We do this so you hit your water target for the day, but leave a little time of little/no water consumption before bed so that you do not wake up in the night to go to the bathroom. Keeping you in that deep sleep zone for optimal recovery, muscle building, health, and fat loss.

#2: CREATING YOUR BAT CAVE

Having a pitch-black room to sleep in is incredibly important as light exposure can disrupt the time it takes for you to fall asleep, as well as the quality of sleep you have once you are asleep. In other words, the hall light should be off, the TV should be off, the blinds should be closed completely, and if you're reading this right now I'm assuming you probably don't have night lights (but if you do, I'd turn them off. The boogey-man is something you're going to just have to face straight on).

You can think about light exposure as being a signal to your body saying "Hey! It's still daylight, it don't need to make any melatonin just yet because the body is probably still working on important stuff!"

This light exposure, even if it is just from your room and not from the sun, all by itself has been demonstrated in solid research to prevent the body from making melatonin, which is the body's primary sleep hormone (**Gooley, J. 2010**). Additionally, this type of light exposure has been directly linked to reducing your sleep quality (**Cajochen, C. 1998**), which then as a by-product will have a ripple effect on everything we have talked about in this book so far.

Powerful, shocking stuff, right? The thought that light exposure alone could create an impact on how you look, how healthy you are, and how you feel on a regular basis is mind boggling. Yet, scientifically validated.

So what's our super-scientific answer to all of this?

Turn the lights off, get in your bat cave, and hope that now that you're doing all these things to optimize your sleep, that damn boogey-man won't come by and keep you up. The guy's a total pest.

But beyond darkness, what else is a bat cave? It's probably pretty cold.

I mean, I've never slept in one, but it's probably a safe assumption, right?

I don't think bats are too worried about having cold feet, especially since there hanging upside down holding on to the cave rocks all night anyhow. Bats also probably can't get portable generators and heaters in there, although I don't have a reference for that.

Moving on, because I actually do have a point to be made here beyond how cool bats are in my own self-dialogue. Sleeping in a slightly colder environment boosts sleep quality and how restful your sleep is. Research shows us that the optimal temperature for your bedroom should be 19 degrees Celsius, or 66.2 Fahrenheit (**Muzet, A. 1984**). You don't need to stick to these numbers exactly like an OCD maniac, but, you should likely opt for a room temperature that is slightly colder than your intuition would want you to do.

If you get under the covers and you're initially pretty chilly, you're probably in a good spot.

#3: UNPLUGGED ELECTRONICS AND MIND

Very simple and very effective. Turn your phone off, turn your computer off, and turn your TV off. No, setting them to "sleep" doesn't count. Turn them completely off and allow them to vacate your mind. Modern times have people incredibly addicted to their technology.

Ever look at your phone when it never even vibrated or made a noise? Yeah, me too.

This pulling effect they have on our minds is a dopamine-reward based system where our brains are actually driven and wired to check our social media feeds to receive a nice little "reward" chemical cascade throughout the brain, mainly with the secretion of a neurotransmitter known as dopamine.

When we do this, we also promote wakefulness chemicals in our body and brain. The body doesn't associate reward signals with "I want to go to bed", we aren't wired to work this way.

Keep these things off so that we can completely release our mind from the "pull" they have on us so we can calm the nervous system down and prime ourselves for a good night's rest (switch on the PNS). We don't need to see updates, work e-mails, or anything that is going to activate our reward pathways or strategic parts of the brain that will engage us in active thinking.

Beyond this active thinking, these electronics and phones provide the light exposure we need to already be avoiding.

If you use your phone as an alarm clock, place it on airplane mode and keep it a good distance away from you. Out of sight, out of mind.

#4: CIRCADIAN RHYTHMS

Our circadian rhythm is often referred to as our "body clock", it is a biological cycle that happens inside of our body that tells us when to sleep and when to wake up; but also plays other physiological roles in appetite regulation, hormone secretion, blood pressure, and many other important functions.

Circadian rhythm comes as a rule on this list due to the importance that is placed upon you in order to solidify and maintain your circadian rhythm. You do this by abiding by one very simple principle:

Go to bed at the same time every night and wake up at the same time every morning.

Accidently stay up late? Get up at the same time anyways. Accidentally sleep in? Go to bed at the same time anyways.

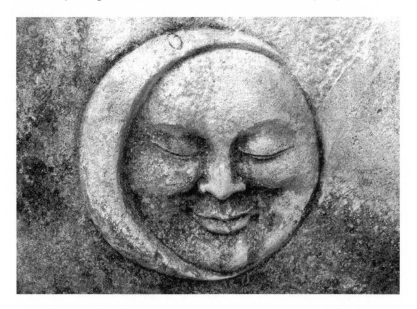

The Sun and Moon, Our Consistent Circadian Rhythm Indicators.

Get in a rhythm of being consistent, this habit will lock your circadian rhythm in place so you can effectively train your body to get tired at the right times of the day to promote optimal sleep.

Then, as time passes and sleep is optimized you will have more energy (as a by-product due to greater sleep length and quality) for your daily work life and training. Beyond this, circadian rhythm regulation is tightly linked to testosterone (anabolic) and cortisol (catabolic) secretion.

The testosterone to cortisol ratio is often used as a biomarker for the anabolic potential somebody has, as well as what their current recovery status is. For example, a greater testosterone to cortisol ratio would represent somebody who is well recovered and has a high potential to build muscle tissue and burn fat.

The circadian rhythm determines when these hormone secretions occur, and to what degree they occur. If you are constantly changing our sleep schedule and habits it is very likely you are not optimizing what hormonal potential you have. Beyond this, for optimal circadian rhythm function it is recommended you get whatever hours you can of sleep before midnight, as opposed to after midnight. Some research (alongside plenty of anecdotal tradition) suggests that every hour of sleep you get before midnight is equivalent to 2hrs of sleep after midnight.

Knowing this, I like to make the recommendation that anywhere between 9 and 10pm is the best bedtime, with 11pm being the absolute latest for optimization.

Research into the consistency of people's' lives have demonstrated that those who have a consistent schedule and lifestyle have greater sleep quality than those who don't (**Monk, T. 200**3), additionally, those with irregular schedules are particularly susceptible to disrupting their sleep quality as it seems sleep quality is very sensitive to changes in your normal scheduling (**Giannotti, F. 2002**).

To put the last nail in the coffin of having a consistent schedule (and perhaps shed light on why shift workers always feel like they are pulling an anchor around), we have seen in research that the sleep quality is higher when you go to bed at your normal times than when you sleep at another time which is off your schedule. For example, if you always sleep from 10pm-6am

every single night, but for one night you deviated from this regular window, the sleep quality you achieve outside of that window would be not as great compared to your normal window and thus result in a reduced sleep quality and recovery status of the body (**Baehr, EK. 2000)**

#5: DEAL WITH YOUR ANXIETY

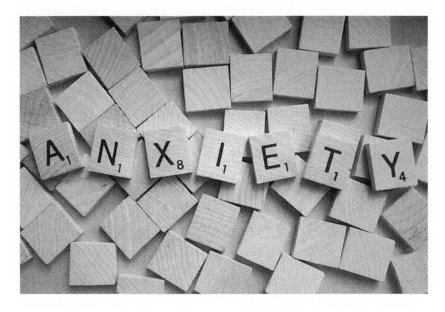

Let it Go

"Man, I wish I could have said 'X' during that argument today. That would have been awesome" "I can't forget to call that guy tomorrow"

"Ok so today I did X, Y, and Z. But by tomorrow at noon I have to have already finished A, B, and C"

"I hope my alarm goes off!"

…Any of these sounds familiar?

I know they did for me, until I used the appropriate tools within the Sequential Shutdown Method to release stress from my life and create the best night's sleep possible every night. Me personally, I am a crazy work/productivity type person. I am always thinking about what projects are currently going on, who I need to contact, and what still needs to be accomplished.

This type of thinking causes the strategic part of the brain to activate and promote wakefulness. Much like the cellphones keep our minds "engaged", not letting go of stressful factors in your life can cause wakefulness as well. Any and all types of pre-bed anxiety, night time planning, or ruminating on the past are going to affect your mind state and alter your ability to fall asleep.

We've all had those nights, your head hits the pillow and your brain won't shut up. It was a deadbeat all day, but for whatever reason now, at 1 o'clock in the morning, it's ready and willing to strategize and think through your problems.

Seriously brain, why do you do this?

The best strategy I have ever come across to eliminate this type of thinking is to write down everything you need to accomplish tomorrow. Write it all out like it is a checklist you are making yourself for tomorrow. Once you write this all out, put it in a place you are 100% guaranteed to see it in the morning. I personally put mine beside the coffee maker, coffee is a part of my morning routine and it's a spot that I am 100% guaranteed to visit first thing upon waking.

You might think this checklist is made to enhance your productivity, and it probably will. Research has demonstrated many times we are much more likely to accomplish goals we physically write down. But this is not the main reason why I want you doing this.

The primary focus here is to create an opportunity for you to release everything in your brain.

Let it all go.

Once everything you need to accomplish tomorrow is on paper, you don't need to remember anything. You can release it completely from your mind and allow yourself to sink into your pillow without a single thing on your mind because everything you need to remember is on paper and in a place you are guaranteed to see tomorrow morning. You'll never miss a beat no matter what, so you can allow yourself to totally let go.

The paper and pen give you freedom, use them.

#6: THE 2HR RULE

Put very simply, put your life on airplane mode 2hrs from the time you go to bed. So if you go to bed at 10pm, your cellphone gets put on airplane mode at 8pm.

No texts.

No e-mails.

No social media checks.

No creeping (not even your ex). No work mail.

No contests.

No anything.

These updates, scrolls, and cybernetic stimulation create activation of certain areas in the brain that promote wakefulness which disrupts the sleep signalling cascade that is supposed to

be winding you down for the day. There are literal chemicals in the body and brain that are in place for sedation, they create feelings of being tired to begin the wind down process for you to optimize your sleep quality. When you disrupt these, you dramatically alter the signalling process and can increase the time it will take for you to fall asleep.

I normally get immediate resistance when I tell clients, friends, or family members of this strategy. The resistance has nothing to do with the scientific research behind the topic (which they conveniently don't check), and everything to do with the fact that people just really don't want to give up their phones.

They are crazy about them and need them by their side. This alone should demonstrate to your how much this affects your brain chemistry before sleep, you know, if all the data on light exposure and brain chemical secretion wasn't enough.

Not to mention, nothing you receive after 8pm will be of any consequence anyways. Any message, work e-mail, or post can wait until the morning. I promise nobody is expecting an immediate answer from you if they message you this late in the day. I personally time block my entire life, all of my friends and family know that I don't answer anything after 8pm. They also know I don't answer anything until 7:30am the next morning, everything is plotted out and organized to maximize my life quality and productivity.

At the same time, I have told them my scheduling so they are already aware and do not have their feelings hurt when I do not reply. You can also include this in your e-mail signature so that everybody is well aware of your scheduling and will not expect an immediate response.

This is done to calm my brain and remove blue light, which we'll talk about next.

#7: BLUE LIGHTS AND THE MORNING SUN

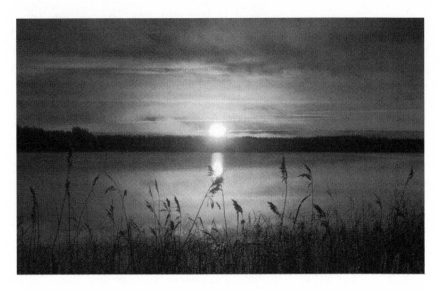

Morning Sunlight

Believe it or not, the light you are exposed to affects your sleep quality in the hours leading up to bedtime. Feeling sleepy is the result of melatonin, a hormone that regulates sleep and provides some sedation effects as well. Bright lights, and specifically blue light, can decrease melatonin production.

To lower your exposure to bright lights and blue light, it is highly recommended to shut your phone and computer down within 2hrs of bedtime.

Notice how rules 2, 3, 6, and 7 all have one thing in common?

A plugged-in mind is an activated mind, and an activated mind is sacrificing sleep quality whether it knows it or not.

If you are completely and hopelessly addicted to your phone and/or computer, which many people are, I would highly recommend you at least install a light reddening app called f.lux, or another option is an app for your phone called Twilight. These apps connect themselves to the sunrise and sunset schedule of your specific location and eliminate the blue light exposure emitted from your phone or computer once sunset has occurred at your geographical location so you are on track with your environment and circadian rhythm.

Of course, you can still activate the areas of the brain that keep you wakeful with strategic thinking, but remember, I said these apps were for the hopelessly addicted. Something is always better than nothing, you bunch of addicts.

On the complete flip side of this, exposure to sunlight in the morning promotes wakefulness early in the day. When you promote wakefulness early in the day you will be promoting an energetic day, but as a byproduct of this you will be ready for bed come night time. Decreasing blue light at night and directly exposing yourself to sunlight upon waking are two of the most powerful things you can do to regulate your circadian rhythm and sleep quality.

Light exposure alone has been demonstrated to improve sleep quality, productivity, and overall well-being (**Viola, AU. 2008).** When you start your day off with a little bit of sun, or if you have difficulty getting sun you can use a full-spectrum lamp with about 10,000 lux power, you're doing your mind, body, and sleeping habits a whole lot of good.

It also doesn't hurt that these apps and the sun are both completely free, the lamp on the other hand might set you back about $25-$40.00 depending on where you live. Devastating, I know.

#8: STIMULANTS AND DEPRESSANTS

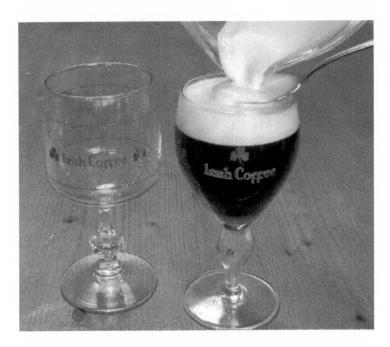

Irish Coffee, the blend of both a stimulant (coffee) and a depressant (alcohol)

Sleep problems affect an estimated 30% of the population, that means every 3rd person you know has self-admitted issues with their sleep and how rested they feel (**Roth, T. 2007**). This is an absolutely huge number.

But do you want to guess what's an even bigger number?

The amount of people who drink alcohol, drink coffee, or smoke tobacco.

Starting with alcohol, I can confidently tell you it is terrible for sleep quality. This is many times misrepresented by people because they feel alcohol helps them get to sleep, which can actually be true.

Alcohol improves most people's ability to **induce** sleep (or you know, pass out), and then it disrupts sleep from there on after. It impairs slow wave sleep and it is a Rapid Eye Movement (REM) suppressant. It will suppress your deep REM sleep. Essentially, your sleep **length** will be identical, but your sleep **quality** will be poor (**Ebrahim, IO. 2013**).

Ever go out partying, and then still sleep a solid 8hrs, but wake up totally exhausted?

Yeah, that's sleep quality vs. sleep length being played out in real life and what REM suppression feels like.

Alcohol has a short half life so a drink at dinner time is normally no problem, but alcohol before bed is a big problem. Getting rid of booze is the first thing on the list if somebody is complaining about sleep. Period.

Somewhat humorous connection between alcohol and sleep here, being awake for 17-19 hours is equal to having a blood alcohol concentration of 0.05 percent as far as performance testing goes — these numbers consider you legally drunk in many states. This sleep deprivation also resulted in 50% slower response times and accuracy measures were even worse than those compared even at that level of alcohol (**Williamson S. 2000**).

After alcohol, we have caffeine use.

Caffeine is totally fine and healthy to have on a habitual basis, one of the biggest myths currently in the industry is the idea that coffee is somehow bad for us, this is absolutely not the case.

In fact, coffee has plenty of research to suggest it has health promoting effects, so this myth couldn't be any more backwards (**Bhatti, SK. 2013**).

But when it comes to our sleep, there are a couple of things to keep in mind. If you are having a pre-workout product or a coffee to jazz-up for your workout at 7pm, this is likely too late and will affect your sleep. The problem here is the fact that caffeine has a **5hr half-life.**

What this means is that half of the active ingredient will be gone after 5hrs, but the other half will still remain. For example, if you have a pre-workout with 200mg of caffeine in it (which is a fairly light pre-workout as far as today's standards go) at 7pm, 100mg of active caffeine substance will still be in your system at midnight. To put it into perspective, 100mg of caffeine is equivalent to a 6oz cup of coffee (standard cup size), which would still be active in your system at midnight.

There are some who are saying "Obviously I'm not going to have a coffee in the PM Dan, the caffeine would keep me up!"

But, you would be surprised. There are plenty of people out there who ask me why they have sleeping issues every night, when they are the ones who also drink coffee at 5pm or later each and everyday. Research is clear in this area that caffeine negatively affects sleep quality, even if you have it 6hrs before bedtime (**Drake, 2013**).

So, if you're one of these people taking stimulants late at night, it's likely best that you save them for the days you can train in the morning and find other, non-sleep alternating ways to get jacked for your session.

Lastly on the stimulant-based sleep structure augmenters, we have nicotine. Nicotine is a potent stimulator of the adrenal cortex, similar to caffeine in this sense. It is also cholinergic, which means it is neurally stimulating for the brain.

REM sleep is a cholinergic phenomenon, and REM sleep is actually an EEG state of waking, this is known as active sleep. The brain is very active during REM sleep, and nicotine induces this same pattern which is disruptive. If you are a habitual smoker, stop smoking from 4pm and on for best for sleep quality and reduced time to fall asleep (**Wetter, DW. 1994**).

#9: DEEP BREATHING TECHNIQUES

Deep breathing is an incredibly underrated activity for stress management, inflammation regulation, and activation of the parasympathetic nervous system. Deep breathing by itself, when done properly, can get you straight into that "rest and digest" state I have continuously alluded to you throughout this book to optimize your recovery and results.

Work with me for a second here. Do not just read, I want you to act.

I want you to pause, clear your mind completely or picture yourself at your personal favorite, most relaxing environment. Mine is sitting on the dock at my Grandparents cottage I visited in Muskoka, Ontario every year as a kid growing up. When I close my eyes and transport myself there, I am immediately in tune with the sounds, sight, and even smell of all of those relaxation cues around me.

Take a moment, and find your place of Zen.

Now that your mind is clear or you have found your place of nirvana, I want you to breath deep into your belly (NOT chest) as deep and as low into your abdomen as you can. Picture the air being brought all the way down to your belly button and then expanding your entire belly. This inhale should take an **easy** 5 seconds, more like 10 seconds.

After this, slowly exhale. Don't let all your air out at once. Let the air go through a small hole in your lips and completely expel all air. Really close your lungs up. They should feel flat as a pancake after your exhale is complete and you should have absolutely zero air left in your chest. This exhale should take an **easy** 10secs.

Repeat this 5-10 times, your mind is in a place of nirvana and we are slowing down your heart rate and breathing by centering our bodies and mind as one.

Do not focus on breathing reps, focus on being present in the moment.

If you live in the future you have anxiety, and if you live in the past you have depression. This exercise, I truly need you to only be here right now. No thoughts, no being, no environment around you, no job, no to-do list today, no social media beckoning you to refresh the screen, no **anything**.

Just you, in your place of happiness, taking deep breaths.

This process will dramatically change your mind state, calm you down, activate the parasympathetic nervous system, and prime both your body and mind your optimal sleep quality (**Jerath, R. 2006**).

Best part of this strategy is that it is completely free of charge, and can be done as often as you need it. Most people who have trouble calming down and falling asleep do best with one of these quick sessions at 5-6pm, and another session around 9pm. I find the sessions earlier in the evening really helps begin the process of calming down, and the later sessions solidifies the sedation and calming effects and allows you to sleep much more peacefully. It's almost as if there is a stress/energy debt to pay in some people, and you can override this all with only one session before bed.

You need one session in the early evening to activate the PNS and send signals to the body that:

"Ok, it's alright to begin calming down now. Work is over, training is over, let's begin the chill-out process"

And then when it comes time for your second round of deep breathing, it dots all the I's and crosses all the T's that were left in the calming down process, leaving you with a completely optimized physiology for rest and rejuvenation.

#10: NAPPING CORRECTLY

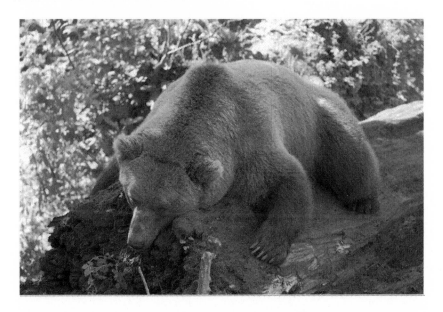

Napping has always results in better gains for my clients, see above for a progress pic*

*Results may vary

Napping can be an effective tool in helping to pay off sleep debt from the previous night(s), but like everything else there is a good way to go about things and a bad way. For example, if somebody were to say:

"Hey, I'm going to start lifting stuff for muscle mass. I don't care about sets or reps or weight, I'm just going to lift"

You would probably be thinking "Hmmm, let me show you some technique and we'll get you on a training program using the scientific principles of training for muscular hypertrophy. After that, let's go through some stuff on your nutrition and recovery"

That seems obvious, right?

We don't just go in the gym and do silly things and then hope to grow.

But then most people don't bat an eye when someone is doing something incorrect with their sleep. No regard to circadian rhythm, no regard to hormone release, no regard to length or quality, no regard to much of anything even though it is a highly-developed science at this point in time.

There are two rules you should follow if you're going to nap throughout the day:

1.   Your body has a natural low in the circadian cycle 12hrs from the midpoint of your sleep cycle. Your midpoint is the exact halfway point of your sleep cycle, so if you slept from 10pm to 6am, your midpoint would be 2am.

So if we are going to nap 12hrs from the midpoint of our sleep cycle, it would be best for us to nap at 2pm. At this point in the day we have a natural energy low (reaching for the afternoon coffee, anyone?) and a nap makes a lot of physiologic sense here to bring us back to life and not disrupt our natural high/low cycles

2.   The nap must be no longer than 30mins in length. Naps longer than 30mins start to induce slow wave sleeping patterns in the

brain which will bring you into a state of deep sleep. This can send the wrong signal to your body because if you habitually do this you will be sending the signal to your body that '2pm is now bedtime' and your body can adjust to this and think that that is when bed time now is based on your actions.

Beyond dysregulating your circadian rhythm, naps longer than 30mins will create a pretty tough sleep inertia to get through. Meaning, you will wake up feeling groggy and slow and not refreshed. Needing to overcome the inertia of the "morning feeling" many of us have before we start waking up to the day. Not exactly my idea of what a good nap in the afternoon should feel like!

In conclusion, if you follow these 10 Rules of Getting the Perfect Night's Sleep I can personally guarantee you will be doing yourself a huge favor by increasing your sleep length and sleep quality dramatically.

The aim of this chapter was to provide you with some further information and research towards the importance of sleep and impact that it has on our physiology, but also offer 10 **EASY** strategies that you can implement right away and are going to make a huge difference in your life.

I hope I have accomplished that goal because ultimately the results you get with your physique and the results that you get with your health depend on how well, or how poorly you sleep.

BULLETPROOF RITUALS FOR SUCCESS

Ritual defined:

A series of actions or type of behavior regularly and invariably followed by someone.

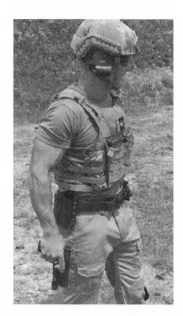

Let me start this chapter off with a short story about one of my clients. My intuition tells me that if you're reading this, you will very likely be able to personally relate to this, or at the very least know somebody close to you in your life that carries this profile.

She was 23 years old and had been on the path towards health and fitness for about 2 years before she decided to send me over an e-mail about personalized coaching.

When she started her journey, she was 5'5" and 163lbs. Her goals revolved primarily around losing some pounds to get to a healthy body weight, and at the same time build a little bit of muscle tissue in some problem areas. She had no desire to be bone-shredded, but wanted to build a booty– she also wanted those "nice shoulders and arms" that "those fit girls have"

I totally got her vision, I've been down this road a million times with female clientele.

Sure thing Jessica, I'll take you on as a client. Let's get after it.

By the time she got to me during her two year journey she had already progressed from a 163lbs starting weight to a present day 145lbs. Without any of my help, she was already much closer to her goals than at the beginning. Progress has clearly been made, but, there was a problem.

That progress came fast and strong until it plateaued **about a year ago**.

Her first year in the gym and developing some healthy new nutrition habits definitely got her from A to B. She lost nearly 20lbs, and was doing the important things much more regularly such as drinking more water, eating the right foods, and making a habit out of exercising at least 3 days a week.

But after the first year, things seemed to stop moving.

She was already following my social media pages and following the tips for awhile before she contacted me, so after a year of stagnation she decided to shoot me over an e-mail and wanted a complete coaching package.

Nutrition, training, and unlimited communication. The whole works.

I ran her through my initial assessments, designed her a customized meal planning and training system, and we were off to the races. Within 3 weeks, she had broken through her plateau and lost another 5lbs, getting her into the high 130's and she was ecstatic.

Phase 1 programming was working, cheers!

But things started to plateau again, so I changed up her training routine to add a little more volume.

I'd like to tell you here that my training routine was the plateau buster that saved the day, but it wasn't. We ran through the new program for about 4 weeks without another drop on the scale.

She got stronger, sure. But this wasn't exactly her goal so she wasn't exactly ecstatic about the past month of hard work.

Of course, this type of situation has her a little frustrated and has me scratching my head just a bit trying to figure out what's going on. But, I'm a coach, and any good coach is a good detective. So, I started digging.

I found out her employment at the hospital was quite stressful, not due to job security but due to petty drama. You know how it is, poor team environments can wear on you overtime.

Beyond this, her shifts at the hospital were disrupting her sleep quality. Working the day shift wasn't so bad, although she still complained of having issues falling asleep and not waking up feeling rested even on the day shift.

The real problem though was with her afternoon shift. It ran until 11pm and she just couldn't seem to wind down afterwards.

BINGO.

THERE'S MY TARGETS.

We have two enormous targets on our hands now, stress and sleep. Two factors that can absolutely railroad your results in the gym and slowly degrade your health. Two factors that also let me know that the Sequential Shutdown Method is going to be **perfect** for this client.

No wonder the augmentation to her training didn't have the desired effect, the over-sympathetic state combined with an under-slept physiology is a recipe for plateaus, no matter how good your training and diet are.

I go back to the drawing board immediately after hearing those details from her and decide that implementing some rituals into her lifestyle is going to be step 1 towards getting through this plateau.

Why a ritual though?

And what kind of ritual would help in this type of scenario?

Well, a ritual is something that you follow each and everyday, no matter what. It's also something that you do automatically. You don't have to force yourself to do a ritual.

As we slowly develop a new technique into a habit, it then ultimately morphs into a personal ritual that will instill long term healthy action-taking towards what's limiting her in her progression at this point (and likely for as long as she remains employed at this hospital).

As far as what kind of ritual we need to implement, we need something that:

• Calms her down to prepare her mind for sleep

• Provides a "turn off" switch for her brain so that when her head hits the pillow, she's ready to sleep and not ready to stay awake all night thinking about random things

• Allow her to quickly and effectively enter a para-sympathetic state (rest and digest, and NOT fight or flight)

• Works in co-ordinance with her schedule and abilities

• Is not too overwhelming to cause even further stress than there already is (worst thing you can do for someone who is stressed is to add a complicated system to make things worse)

• Will work to both de-stress her, and allow the proper hormonal cascades to begin kicking in for optimal sleep length and sleep quality to get her progress humming along again

That's a tall order, but a well-designed ritual can work wonders. Here's exactly what I had her do:

1. Listen to your favorite music on your iPod on the way home

from work

2.   When you get home, write down six things that you need to accomplish tomorrow

3.   Once you have written down six things you need to accomplish tomorrow, write down three things that you are grateful for that happened today

4.   5mins of deep breathing exercises of your choice

5.   5mins of complete silence

What's important here is what these acts do towards your physiology, and why the order in which you execute this ritual is prescribed for a reason. It also doesn't hurt that all of them are 100% free of charge to you, that's assuming you have some sort of music device. I think my assumptions safe that if you are reading an eBook, you likely aren't a caveman and are familiar with these new fandangled "iPods" or "cellphones" that the whipper-snappers on your lawn keep carrying around.

By the way, Jessica?

She dropped an additional 8.1lbs within the next 4-weeks after I prescribed this ritual with absolutely zero changes made to her training or nutritional strategy. Of course this made me look like some sort of genius, but that's only because the vast majority of people overlook just how important sleep is towards the equation reaching your physique and health goals.

Without this ritual or my guidance, she may have done what most everybody else does – try and eat a lot less and while doing a little more cardio after each workout. Sure, this could work.

But for how long?

How long can you sustain that? Especially given that this was an everyday person just looking to look and feel better, and not training for a bodybuilding or fitness show. People need sustainable options; pre-contest dieting and training is not sustainable.

I think the much more approachable and maintainable strategy here would be to continue eating the same amount of food, but improve your overall stress tolerance and sleep quality through well-designed rituals. Let's talk a bit about why I did what I did, and cover each aspect of the ritual:

Listen to your favorite music on the way home from work: Very simple, but very powerful stuff here. It's a complete shift in mindset without having to put any effort into it. If I said to

her "think happy thoughts on the way home from work" like some sort of kumbaya wacko, she probably would have said "Yeah I'll do that", and maybe she would have gave it a try. But probably not. Telling somebody to "think happy" is comparable to telling somebody "Hey! Stop being stressed!"

Sure, they are good ideas. **But how!?**

Offering strategies as vague as that are unlikely to work in the long term. But, being instructed by your coach to listen to your favorite music?

Sure, you don't have to tell me twice!

The very act of listening to your favorite music allowed her to get into a positive stress-free mind state and leave the petty drama and stress at work behind her.

A quiet drive home would likely lead to her reminiscing about something negative that happened that day, or care more about the stress of driving.

I take the radio out of the equation, because let's face it, the radio sucks. I also take the silence out of the equation, because that's not a guaranteed positive switch. This leaves me to instruct her bring her iPod and leave it in her car, and play her music on the way home to melt away the stress.

In other client scenarios, I have used a similar strategy to this but actually have the client listen to stand up comedy routines. The act of smiling and laughing creates incredible cascades of chemicals in the body which totally oppose the stress hormones that keep us awake at night and create the negative impacts of a chronically elevated SNS (remember, our goal in these later hours is to switch "off" the SNS).

So if you're not a music kind of person or if you're looking to switch things up once in awhile, comedy does a phenomenal job of turning your entire mood around and allow you to deflect any negativity or stress away from your life.

Write down six things that you have to do tomorrow: This is one that has helped me immensely in my life within both the productivity and stress management realms, and is one of the most powerful tools in the entire ritual towards improving in your sleep quality.

How it works is you think about anything that you have to do tomorrow and just brain dump it down on paper:

•   Laundry

•   Dentist appointment at 4pm

•   E-mail your client back

•   Renew your licence

•   Workout at 7am

- Finish that assignment

- Clean your office space

- Get groceries

- Meet your friend for coffee at 11am

- Contact your accountant about this years upcoming tax return

- Yell at the phone company for your most recent bill

- Etc...

Some of these things might look silly to you, but, there is real magic here. First off, there is good research out there demonstrating that you are much more likely to complete a task if you write it down, so you get a little productivity boost out of this (**Matthews, G. 2015**).

But, what was most impactful towards Jessica here was how stress-free this makes your life. You now have everything you need to do tomorrow on paper, **you're free now – you don't have to remember ANYTHING.**

Everything you need to do is a part of the physical world now, you can release all of those thoughts and all of that anxiety towards hoping you don't forget what you need to do or if you will be late for any of them.

Release it all, let it all go.

This here is the essence of the 5th rule towards getting the perfect night's sleep. Now you can go to bed with supreme confidence and zero anxiety because when you wake up tomorrow you're going to see your list and knock every last item down. No stress, no anxiety, no trying to remember anything; just execution.

This brain release creates a powerful relaxation effect before you go to bed because you have the feeling that you have your life under control. It's ok for you to fall asleep, because you're 100% prepared for tomorrow and you won't forget a single thing. I noted within the ritual to only write down six things, but it should be seen as a minimum, and not an absolute number. In other words, make sure you write down six things, but if you have more to do keep the list going. Get it all out of your mind, this should be a full brain dump.

Write down three things that you were grateful for today: One of the best things somebody can do for themselves is purchase a small journal and pen and use those to create their very first grateful log.

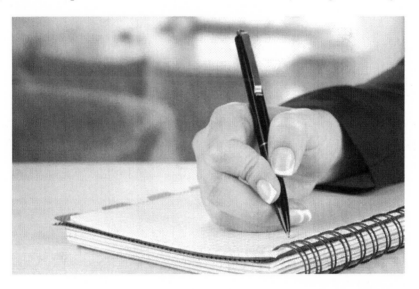

I ask my clientele very often to do this and the ones who follow through find out some cool things about what they truly value in life, but also report a massive improvement in their quality of sleep.

Have you ever sprained your ankle or broken a bone in your leg and been out of commission and off your feet until it heals?

Then you know how grateful feels, you become so grateful for your ability to walk/run and your pain-free movement when the healing is done.

Or even the smaller things in life, one time I had to get my car fixed and the shop held onto it for almost three weeks. You don't realize how dependant are a car to live a convenient life until you lose your car for three weeks. Man, was I ever happy to have my beat up Civic back. It turns out having your Mom drive you to work everyday doesn't go unnoticed by the guys at work, they'll let you know that too.

Being grateful for what you have in your life creates a very calm and positive mind state. It helps you view your personal world in a positive light before going to sleep and helps reduce what I call "night time chaos" where an individual's mind races all over the map for hours until they are able to finally fall asleep.

Being grateful, being positive, and being calm all lead to a dramatic improvement in the quality of your sleep but also the time it takes in order for you to fall asleep. Every sentence you write down should begin with:

"Today, I was grateful for..."

And you should fill out a minimum of three, but of course there is no restriction here as to how many things you can be grateful for in a single day (Unless you're Ned Flanders, in which case you should probably cap it off around five hundred and call it a night).

It's very easy for us to be negative about our situations or experiences. For example, if you go to a local restaurant and receive good service. I'm sure you had a good time and some good food, but you're probably unlikely to remember this or go home and immediately tell your friends and family about it.

On the other hand, if you go to this same restaurant and receive terrible service, you are highly likely to remember everything very vividly, tell your friends and family not to go there, and allow it to bother you for the rest of your day.

Negativity just seems to magnify itself in our worlds, take a moment before bed to reinstate your positivity, happiness, and gratitude. We could all use some.

5mins of deep breathing exercises: Before getting into this, I want you to place your right hand on your chest and place your left hand on your stomach.

Now, take two deep breaths in. Inhaling as much as you possibly can, and exhaling as much as you possibly can.

Which hand moved more?

The one on your chest? Or the one on your stomach?

If your right hand moved more, you're likely in the large majority of the population who now breath habitually within their chest. This isn't your fault, most of us aren't even aware of it, breathing is just an automatic thing right?

Well, it takes one to know one.

sigh - stands up.

"I'm Dan Garner, and I'm a chest breather"

Sits back down and looks at his shoes

This used to be me, in the dark, **dark** days of chest breathing my way through life. An intervention was forced upon me after reading Dr. Sapolsky's work. I e-mailed him in 2012 to let him know his work released me of chest breathing anonymous. I'll let you know when he replies.

Thankfully, I'm no longer a chest breather. Why did I change my breathing though? What's wrong with chest breathing?

And why on earth would I want my client to change her breathing for 5mins before bed? Flashback to rule #9 of getting the perfect night's sleep (deep breathing exercises).

Chest breathing is the exact **opposite** of this.

Chest breathing is a known trigger/perpetuator of the sympathetic (fight or flight) response. Chronically triggering this branch of our nervous system as you have already learned throughout this eBook in great detail can lead to chronic stress, poor sleep quality, reduced sleep length, and plenty of other less than awesome physiological effects that lead to us being fractions of what we could otherwise be.

Second, it sets off a rhythmic cascade of improper muscle activation. The chest, intercostals, neck, and upper back aren't supposed to be primary muscles involved in our breathing pattern. With habitual use, this can lead to an unhealthy posture and muscle compensation issues.

Lastly, when you're a chest breather you're also a shallow breather. If you're a shallow breather you are not effectively transferring oxygen to your muscle cells through your blood as you otherwise could be if you were doing deep diaphragmatic breathing (stomach breathing).

You ever see a UFC or boxing fight?

In between rounds the experienced fighters are never frantically trying to breath really fast through their chest. Instead, they slow their breathing right down and take deep belly breaths until the bell rings again.

This lowers their heart rate and delivers more oxygen to their muscles so they recover faster, and they ready to rock again. Take notice next time you watch a professional fight. They'll sit on the stool, immediately take their mouth guard out, straighten up their posture, and take deep belly breaths while their coach instructs them on the next rounds game plan. I like this example, although I'm pretty sure I'd be happy to take any excuse in order to watch a fight.

Fact is, most of us spend all day in a heightened sympathetic state due to road rage, conversation anxiety, work, drama, relationship issues, noise pollution, your boss on your ass, money problems, frustration with our fitness goals, family issues, problems with our confidence, the never-ending house projects, bills, – you name it, most of us are walking around with some form of stress **all the time**.

As Bessel Van Der Kolk famously said, "The body keeps the score"

Meaning, each of these stressors creates a physical insult on our body. Don't forget the very first thing I said in this book, the body and mind are completely interconnected. **Your body keeps the score**, all these stressors put one up on the scoreboard of damage to our physiology.

In the short term, stress can be a manageable and even healthy thing.

But over the long term, that scoreboard starts getting imbalanced and you start falling apart.

Deep breathing triggers immediate activation of our parasympathetic system, allowing the body to turn on its machinery to recover properly and effectively manage the stressors in our lives.

5mins is all you need here in almost all cases.

Using the feedback from your hands, I would like you to sit on the edge of a chair with a very straight posture (no need to sit on the floor with your thumbs and index fingers touching and go full yogi here) and place one (or both) of your hands on your belly. This physical touching on your belly can bring a greater state of awareness towards where you should be bringing your air in and what muscles you should be activating in order to breath properly.

From here, close your eyes and take the deepest inhales you possibly can. Use the muscles in your stomach to push your stomach outwards while doing your best to have a still upper body and calm mind. When you exhale, just let the belly return to normal as you learn these new techniques.

Repeat these deep breaths consecutively for 5mins and do your best to keep a clear mind.

5mins of complete silence: Complete silence of the body and mind is becoming more and more important as our society becomes more and more noisy, fast-paced, and over stimulated by social media.

I want you to engage in silence with a purposeful mindset. Purposeful silence.

We aren't just "not talking". We are silencing our mind, completely relaxing our body, and offering us an opportunity for a chance at enlightenment.

Most people allow their lives to be one long chain of clutter, it's always one thing after the next and during any downtime there is still constant stimulation through cellphones, TV, social media, and advertisements hidden around every corner.

Purposeful silence is silence with a purpose, we are eliminating stimulation and "noise" from our mind to gain clarity on ourselves and to enter a state of relaxation that otherwise could not be reached if we were exposed to the many addictive "pulls" life has to offer.

More than anything I want this to be a time for you to let go of your compulsive need to constantly be thinking about something. This is a moment where you are truly in the present, there is no future and you have no past. All of your worries are evaporated because you are only right here, right now.

This is often referred to as just **being.**

Not thinking, not planning, not doing, just being.

Imagine yourself inhaling positivity and calmness, and exhaling negativity, worry, and stress with every breath. Enjoy this purposeful silence, this time is yours. Just be.

What to do:

• The first step is to prepare your mindset and expectations. It is incredibly harder than you expect to try and think about absolutely nothing. Prepare your mind to be very calm, but if your mind wanders you must not get frustrated. Simply come back into a state of nothingness without judgement of yourself for getting off track

• Find a comfortable place to sit and sit with a good posture. Do not lie down, you must sit

• Close your eyes

• Take slow, deep breaths throughout this time. It doesn't have to be the deep breathing intensity that we utilize in the deep breathing ritual, just ensure you aren't chest breathing would be the only note here

• If you have a relentless influx of thoughts or emotions, it may help you to concentrate on a mantra. "Breathe in…….. Breathe out" repeated throughout the process can help, although the ideas for mantras are endless

• "Breathe in positivity……. Breathe out negativity"

• "Inhale………. Exhale"

• Or the classic "Ohmmmmmmmmmm"

• Turn your phone completely off And that's it.

There's no perfect way to approach silence, whatever works best for you to achieve a state of **being** is going to be the best option for you. Me personally, I do 5mins of silence on the edge of my office chair with all of my electronics in the room off and I also wear earplugs during this time so that I have as little stimulation as humanly possible.

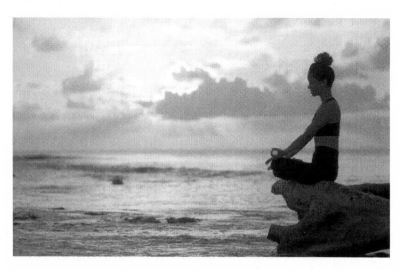

Despite most people's preferences, my office is actually a place where I am completely and totally comfortable and can reach a state of complete relaxation. I love it in there.

I highly recommend you choose a place you are already totally and completely comfortable in to do your own silent treatment.

In the beginning, this may be hard for you. Especially if you have ADHD, or, OCD tendencies to looking at your phone or other distractions. But, if you keep trying you will begin to love this. My 5mins of silence is honestly one of my favorite moments of the day now, and clients who stick with this continuously all report to me incredible rates of happiness and improvement.

Just remember, don't just sit in silence. Sit in purposeful silence.

Powerful stuff, right?

You can now see how the ritual I designed for the original case study I told you about, Jessica, had such a profound effect on her body and life without me even touching her training or nutrition at the time. It looked simple on paper, but here's what we accomplished:

1.   Listen to your favorite music on the way home

a.   Calmed the mind

b.   Created a positive mind state

c.   Forgot the stress of work and stress of traffic

d.   Switched off anxiety and the SNS

2.   Write down six things that you need to accomplish tomorrow

a.   Calmed the mind

b.   Enhanced productivity in all areas of her life

c.   Reduced anxiety

d.   Reduced night-time thinking/remembering

e.   Allowed for an empty mind to go to bed with

f.   Enhanced organization

g.   Improved professionalism

3.   Write down three things that you are grateful for

a.   Calmed the mind

b.   Created a positive mind state

c.   Reminder of what's important in life

d.   Switches on the PNS

e.   Engages the mind to remember what's positive, instead of just what is negative

4.   5mins of deep breathing

a.   Calmed the mind

b.   Switch from a sympathetic to a parasympathetic state

c.   Teaches you proper breathing mechanics for muscle oxygenation

d.   Improves muscle contraction patterning

e.   Improves recovery and blood flow

f.   Lowers the heart rate

5.   5mins of silence

a.   Calmed the mind

b.   Created a positive mind state

c.   Perpetuate and "cement in" the parasympathetic state

d.   Enter deep relaxation

e.   Train the body to resist being stuck in the past or in the future

f.   Train the body to resist the many "pulls" around us and allow us to just be

g.   Create "Me time" removed from the many stimulations of society

This all creates the perfect storm for a dramatically improved sleep length and sleep quality; which will directly affect the results you get out of the gym. Whether that be health based, fat loss, or muscle gain, sleep and parasympathetic activation will help you in all three areas **dramatically**.

Not to mention, this ritual takes less than 20mins a night so the return on time invested makes it an absolute no-brainer.

If you want the best results out of your efforts in the gym and you want to create a healthy body and mind while you're at it, begin to incorporate one or all of these rituals today. Take action now to start changing your life like so many clients of mine have before you.

Pick one, or all, and just do it.

I promise your life will improve dramatically because of it.

THE SEQUENTIAL SHUTDOWN METHOD

I would like to tell you I was in a lab coat at midnight laughing like a madman while lightning struck dramatically in the background when I originally discovered the SSM, but, like most things in this book, you'll discover I boringly and slowly put things together over time by coming across new data and allowing the process to prove itself through periodic experimentation and implementation. Sexy, I know.

Through dozens of clients like Jessica, I knew the rituals were a mainstay in my coaching arsenal. Anything that repeatedly produces results within a client's psychology, parasympathetic nervous system, productivity, stress reduction, anxiety, and improvement in sleep length and sleep quality is a damn good tool to hold on to. This becomes especially true since the rituals will likely net you no financial loss, or at most a few bucks for a journal.

The rituals didn't always begin the way in which I articulated with Jessica, I toyed and manipulated them across many different clients and eventually ended up sticking with the ritual guidelines I outlined above as they just seemed to work the best across the board for the wide variety of demographics that I work with on a daily basis.

Understanding the rituals' importance, we also have to take into consider all ten rules in order to create the perfect night's sleep. The thing with these rules is that they are exactly that, rules. I don't want to sound like that school teacher you used to hate, but, rules are made for a reason.

When it comes to your sleep, violating just one of these rules can throw all of your efforts off.

Following nine of the ten rules and some rituals but stay on your phone all night? Sorry, research suggest you're decreasing your melatonin.

Following nine of the ten rules but keep drinking water late into the night? Sorry, nocturia has been demonstrated multiple times over in the research to reduce sleep quality.

Think you're slick by creating the bat cave, but don't go to bed and wake up at the same time everyday? Sorry, your circadian rhythm is dysfunctional and this lack of routine reduces sleep quality.

I'd honestly like to continue here and hold on to the jerk teacher role a little longer, but I think you get the point.

Moving forward, let's define something first:

se•quen•tial

sə'kwen(t)SHəl

1.   forming or following in a logical order or sequence. - "a series of sequential steps"

2.   Performed or used in sequence.

The SSM is all in place for a reason, the best case scenario is that you follow this sequence in the order I articulate it for the best results you can get. Here's how it breaks down:

Step 1

Ensure you and your environment are following the 10 rules for engineering the perfect night's sleep. If you're stuck at where to start, one of the best methods in which you can determine what will have the greatest impact on you here is to give yourself a grade out of 10 for each and every rule. The two rules that you scored the lowest on are likely the two biggest reasons you're not maximizing your sleep.

Step 2

Follow the Bullet-proof Rituals. Yes, I want you to follow all of them. But, if you must try and "hack" this (I hate that term) and you only want to pick a few, the silence, gratitude, and to-do list are your non-negotiables. If you want the full effect of the SSM, do everything in this book, all ten rules and all the rituals. But, if you want to shorten things down; find the two rules you score the lowest in for the 10 rules, and then follow the silence, gratitude, and to-do list rituals.

Step 3

Incorporate well-researched supplementation to maximize the process. Below is an entire section I have dedicated to the book on proper supplementation as I have seen through experience how impactful proper supplementation at the proper time can be towards getting the best night's sleep and getting a kick ass physique. I have created both basic and advanced protocols for you to follow below and have put them all through an intense screening process where they had to have excellent data on them, as well as they had to have **already created amazing results with my current clientele**. These are protocols that I utilize on a daily basis with my clients, and can be the real catalyst which sends you over this plateau and into the next world of gaining progress each and every workout.

And that's it. That's the SSM. It might look simple since it's a three step protocol, but that's the beauty of it. Don't overcomplicate the process. Do what works, and make it happen. Besides, if you think the SSM looks simple, I'd like to refer you to the dozens of scientific references throughout this book that guided and supported those steps as well as my personal client rosters results you saw before purchasing this program.

This stuff works, and this is the sequence you must follow in order to shutdown the body and prepare for fat loss and growth.

10 rules? Check.

Rituals? Check.

Advanced supplementation protocols? Let's get into it...

PROTOCOL SECTION

Before we dive into what supplementation strategies are relevant for the Eat, Sleep, Burn program – it's important we first go through an education process behind how I came about choosing each supplement and what "tools of knowledge" you can take with you moving forward for the rest of your life that will allow you to more accurately choose the correct and safe supplements for your goals and ultimate vision.

UNDERSTANDING SUPPLEMENTS

Supplements play an interesting role in the health and fitness industry. There are folks who are completely all for them, and on the other side there are people who are completely against them.

What I try to do here with the Eat, Sleep, Burn system is look for truth, which is the only way in which I can provide you with the 100% best service possible and ensure all the money you spend on your supplementation goes towards true investments in your goals, and not in wasting your time, money, and efforts. Unfortunately, a lot of people waste far too much money on useless supplements these days. On top of this, it's hard to even tell what you're taking anymore.

What do I mean by that?

Well, many products on today's shelves are actually spiked with substances that shouldn't even be in there, on top of this, 15-25% of supplements contain **banned substances** that aren't even on the label (**Geyer, 1999** + **HFL, 2007**.)

People who are ignorant to this fact take unknown substances that are having god knows what effect on their body.

Trust me, it takes one to know one.

Before I chose this as a career path and dove full-time into the real research behind these compounds, I wasted thousands of dollars on supplements that never gained me an ounce of muscle, or lose me any weight besides the weight in my wallet.

The amount of testosterone boosters and N.O. products I bought in my teenage years are laughable, and I'm not even kidding, probably thousands of dollars we are talking here.

Then as time passes, you come to realize the only way one can find the truth on a certain topic is to review the current body of scientific evidence and make recommendations based on what has been proven to work through dozens of clinical trials; and **NOT** marketing campaigns.

As you probably know by now, there are a lot of good supplements out there, **but there are also a lot more useless ones.**

Before prescribing supplemental protocols to my clientele I run them through a checklist that was taught to me by the brilliant people over at Precision Nutrition.

1. Is there a chance your diet is currently deficient in this nutrient?

2. Am I targeting the correct system and/or tissue that is necessary for improvement with my goals?

3. Does the current body of evidence show that this nutrient not only works consistently, but is also safe for long term consumption?

Supplements can be a double-edged sword, some are great for you, but others can do more harm than good. Then there's the group of nutrients that are completely neutral, neither good nor bad for you; unless you take your financial savings into consideration.

If the nutrient passes all three of the above tests and has a reasonable amount of data behind it, then it becomes approved for use within the Eat, Sleep, Burn program to enhance your results and bring you from good, to great.

Let's start off with question #1: **Is there a chance your diet is currently deficient in this nutrient?**

Unfortunately, due to today's standards in food quality and general knowledge in nutrition, the overwhelming majority of us who do not supplement are subject to several different vitamin and mineral sub-clinical and/or clinical deficiencies. These base nutrients are absolutely vital to the success in any of your health and fitness goals. Without the basics, you have a much greater possibility of plateauing within your current goals and sacrificing your current state of health.

Vitamins and minerals have to be there for everybody, but they especially have to be there for the active population who deplete and utilize them more often to support progress and

performance. I'm looking at you person who is reading this program! Yeah, you! You're vitamin and mineral status in the body and intake through the diet is dramatically important and ensures you have the appropriate co-factors for success in actions such as energy production, detoxification, and hormone creation.

Let's take magnesium for example, it is estimated that less than 50% of the American population gets adequate magnesium per day through their daily diet (**Marier, JR. 1986**). When you have a look at magnesium's functions (it has over 300 biochemical functions in the body by the way) you quickly find out magnesium:

- Improves quality of sleep

- Improves brain function

- Raises testosterone levels

- Maximizes protein synthesis

- Decreases inflammation

- Improves bone health

- Improves insulin sensitivity

- Detoxifies the stress hormone cortisol

- Improves bowel movements and digestive related disorders

- Aids in bringing down abdominal fat and central obesity

- Is necessary for muscular contraction

- Aids in the prevention of cramps and muscle tears

- Regulates sodium and potassium in and out of the muscle cell

Given that less than 50% of the American population is low on magnesium and this includes those who are inactive and don't deplete magnesium as often as the active population (you!), it would take an obscene and unsustainable amount of vegetables and raw nuts to get your levels just back up to adequate, let alone optimal. To provide some greater context towards magnesium needs for the active population, Nielson et al demonstrated within their research that the active population requires an estimated 20% greater magnesium intake per day (**Nielson, FH. 2006**).

You doing the math?

Less than 50% get their intake in per day, and it doesn't even take into account that many people within that population are also depleting it 20% faster as well.

Magnesium levels = Rock bottom

All those functions mentioned above? Sleeping on the job!

Most importantly, magnesium is just one mineral, and look at all it is involved in. Think about the many functions of all the other minerals and how you could be optimizing your results at this point.

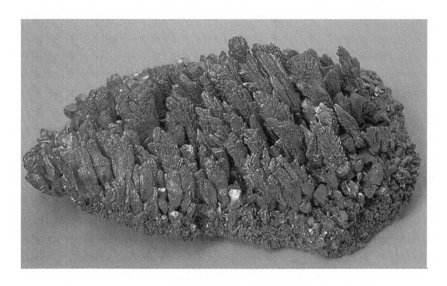

Magnesium, get it in ya!

Do you think a deficiency in magnesium could hold you back in your goals and may be a limiting factor towards progressing to where you want to be?

I can tell you right now, **YES**.

A single deficiency in any vitamin or mineral can 100% hold you back in your progress.

Knowing this, think about the realistic scenario in which you may have sub-optimal levels of several nutrients?

It would be detrimental to any health and fitness endeavour you set out on, no matter how good your training program was.

Which is why it made it to our questionnaire criteria for this highly specific and quality controlled Eat, Sleep, Burn program. If the odds are high you are deficient in a given nutrient, it's a smart idea to begin to supplement to ensure you are covering your bases from what your diet is likely falling short in.

Remember, this becomes even more true for the physically active population. They need even more of these vitamins and minerals on a daily basis, it's no mistake why you see my elite NFL, NHL, UFC, and MLB athletes on a year-round supplement regime to cover their needs.

Certain vital nutrients are depleted through exercise and also utilized to build muscle, burn fat, and remove fatigue producing by-products from the body, four things you will constantly be doing throughout the duration of this program.

Moving on to #2: **Am I targeting the correct system and/or tissue that is necessary for improvement with my goals**?

Supplements work through different pathways and feedback mechanisms in the body to affect the given tissue or system you are trying to target. When taking a supplement, always ask yourself if it is something that is going to positively affect the certain tissue or system that can help you with your goals. In this case, supporting your body composition goals, sleep length, or sleep quality.

For example, creatine improves anaerobic power output and anaerobic work capacity (**Lamontagne-Lacasse, M. 2011** + **Juhasz, I. 2009**). So, for creatine to be beneficial, you would be best off being involved in some sort of anaerobic activity. Anaerobic activities would include weightlifting, sprinting, all martial arts, hockey, hammer throw, etc. Basically any sport that demands explosive, high intensity movement.

Knowing this, it wouldn't make much sense for a marathon runner or a rower to take creatine, given that both of their sports primarily utilize the aerobic system for energy substrate use and not the anaerobic system.

So, even though creatine does have research proven benefits that anybody or any company could reference, it wouldn't have any major benefit for these two above mentioned aerobic sports. Carrying around the additional water weight from creatine while simultaneously not supporting your energy system sport-specific demand doesn't sound like a good trade-off to me. This is a good example showing that although a supplement might be good and have legitimate positive evidence, it will have a totally neutral effect on you because you're not the

target audience for the given nutrient as it won't affect the tissues or energy systems you desire.

You need to understand the demands of your activity and match up the appropriate meal plan and supplementation system for it to work optimally.

Another example on understanding supplemental pathways is the case for Vitamin D in the production of testosterone. Vitamin D plays a role in the production of steroid hormones and studies have shown that men supplementing with Vitamin D over the course of a year increase testosterone levels significantly (**Pilz, S. 2011**)

Having said that, anecdotal reports suggest Vitamin D should be taken in the morning due to its effect on decreasing sleep quality if taken too close to bedtime. This makes sense given the fact that your body associates Vitamin D with sun exposure and if the sun is out giving the body Vitamin D, your body won't respond with making proper sleep hormones because it thinks you're out in the sun and that it is daytime.

Just think about what your internal clock must think when it is 9pm and you just took a 5000IU bomb of sunlight into your body?

Here's the long-term problem, as we discussed at length above, impairing sleep quality has a detrimental effect on testosterone and anabolic hormone production, among many other things you have learned about so far within this book. So, taking Vitamin D for increasing testosterone makes sense, but taking it close to bedtime negates anything you were initially trying to do due to its negative impact on sleep.

Smart in theory, counterproductive in execution.

Pick your supplements wisely and understand the affect they have on your physiology so you can determine if it is worth your time, or not worth anything to you. The main pathways in which workout performance and body composition based supplements work through are:

- Boosting adrenal output

- Increase muscle recovery

- Alter muscle pH

- Stimulate protein synthesis

- Increase anabolic hormones

- Decreased appetite signalling

- Increase fatty oxidation capacity

- Promote healthy homeostasis of targeted systems

- Enhance aerobic (or) anaerobic energy metabolism

I have you 100% covered within this Eat, Sleep, Burn program for pathway maximization to improve all aspects of muscle building, fat loss, health, and performance. Do what I say, and you'll make progress.

But take this knowledge lesson with you for life. It's your body, always ensure you know what system and/or tissue you are trying to affect with the supplementation you are purchasing to maximize your results-- and the weight of your wallet of course.

The last question we must answer prior to the supplemental recommendations for the Eat, Sleep, Burn program is #3: **Does the current body of evidence show that this nutrient works and is safe for consumption?**

This is the sure-fire way to guarantee no money is being wasted and that what you are taking is supporting your goals in muscle building, fat loss, performance, and overall improved health profile. And, you know, doesn't contain foreign objects or banned substances. That's always good.

There are tens of thousands of research papers available on supplementation alone and their effects on the human body and performance. My job is to evaluate the research, keep the good, throw out the bad, and ensure I can confidently stand behind my recommendations.

Not just through personal experience but also through **scientific evidence** as well.

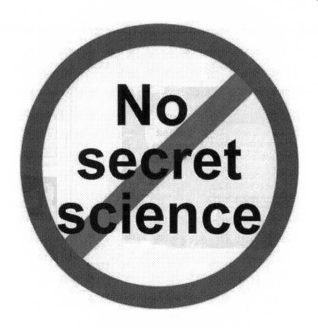

If you haven't noticed yet, this book is heavily referenced for a reason. Real science brings real results. The "why" behind the plan is available to everyone who is curious enough to check out the data.

Although it should be noted here that all governing bodies are different regarding their lists of approved and disapproved substances for sport. Always be sure to check with your governing body of competition to ensure everything you are taking isn't against any of the rules if you

are currently a competing athlete. Some leagues have a very different set of rules than other leagues, and a league can even have varying regulations based only upon certain geographical regions. Always play on the safe side and match everything up with the provided lists of approved substances, these are very easy to get access to.

To make the recommendations found below, not only did the research have to be of a very high quality, but there also needed to be plenty of it. A big lesson here, don't take the research from one study to mean anything. There are tons of studies out there, many of which totally contradict each other. Supplement companies love to jump on the results of one specific study, reference it in their marketing and then sell as much as they can. One study doesn't mean anything, even if it looks promising. There should be lots of available evidence demonstrating a positive effect and a sound research consensus between top authorities in the field.

Beyond this, I have experience with these compounds and have worked with over a thousand clients in my career. Research is important, absolutely. But, experience is equally important.

You can't just talk the talk, you also have to walk the walk. My recommendations below reflect a blend of experience based knowledge of what I know works, as well as purely evidence-based nutrients with very well known objective data behind them.

BUILDING THE FOUNDATION

A staple supplement stack is a stack that is run regardless of the current training phase or goal. It covers all the base nutrients required for optimal bodily function and provides you a foundation to build off of.

You can think about it like building a house.

A house cannot be built just on the ground, it requires a concrete foundation on the bottom. That's what your staple stack is, a concrete foundation that allows you to add things to it. If this foundation wasn't here, the house would collapse. Likewise, if these staples aren't here, you're focusing your financial and physical investments into the wrong areas. It is only after you have built a foundation that you can personalize and optimize your supplement stacks with some more specific options that have a greater targeted effect on your physiology.

Often, the more specific protocol options have way cooler looking advertising and marketing strategies.

Do you know why?

Because it's a much harder sell.

The staple options have the best and most compelling evidence behind them, they don't need a full page ad with a dude flexing to sell them. Everybody knows they are already good. Just like in the grocery store, there are no neon signs or fancy packaging around the vegetables articulating all of the effects they have on your longevity, disease prevention, health, and body composition. Everybody already knows they are the best for you, no selling required.

Whereas lots of the fancier supplement options currently on the market hardly do anything for your body. The reality is, when recommending supplementation to the general public to have a meaningful impact on improving their sleep and performance, there is only a handful of options that have the required data in order for me to confidently recommend them.

But I'll say once again, **YOU NEED THAT FOUNDATION FIRST.**

A proper foundation for anybody interested in improving their overall health, strength, conditioning, performance, and sleep quality should include excellent sources of:

- Multivitamins and minerals

- Fish oil

- Magnesium

- Vitamin D3

- Probiotics BioTrust Pro X10

These nutrients provide the ground floor in which your more specific sleep or performance stacks can work off of, they are a "must have" for the intensely active population looking for serious physique transformation. Through following the criteria in this manual and through years of experience working with thousands of athletes, here are my top picks for each supplement:

Fish Oil - Biotrust OmegaKrill 5X

Multivitamin

Vitamin D3

Magnesium

Probiotics: Biotrust Pro-X10

Before scrolling down and only looking at the more advanced stacks options, I would urge you to incorporate these 5 products **habitually** into your routine before adding anything else.

Additionally, although not considered "foundational" due to the availability in the diet. I highly recommend picking up a whey protein isolate and a carbohydrate powder to meet both your post-workout and throughout the day energy and recovery needs. Whey and liquid carbohydrates both have a tremendous amount of positive research behind them at this point in time, which is why it needs to be mentioned before moving on if getting the greatest

transformation possible is something you want to accomplish. Here are my favorite products:

EAT, SLEEP, BURN: ADVANCED PROTOCOLS

Within the protocol section, I am already under the assumption that you understand the importance of the foundation and that they are already in practice. The foundation stack not only partakes in all of the below protocols, but also **enhances their efficacy**. Meaning, all five foundation products would be added to every protocol in every scenario. I don't care how you do it, just get them in there.

Immune boosting protocol:

1.   Biotrust Metabo Greens– 1 scoop, 1-2x daily in water.

2.   Vitamin C – 1-2x caps daily with food.

3.   Garlic – 600mg, 2-3x daily with food.

4.   Glutamine – 1 teaspoon upon waking, 1 teaspoon before bed

NOTES: The immune system is wildly important for long term success in the game of physique transformation and optimal performance. When you train hard, whether in the gym or in your sport, it is your immune system that is responsible for repairing your body from that exercise so that you can come back stronger and better next time. I reserve this protocol for athletes who tend to get sick often, or, during the later stages of their in-season where immune function tends to drop due to lots of travelling in combination with a large training volume. Think about how often athletes get sick or really feel "the grind" of the season right before or during playoffs, this really helps eliminates that. If you get worn down due to a variety of stressors (training, travel, shift work, etc) then this is a stack for you.

Muscle building protocol:

1.   **<u>Creatine Monohydrate</u>** – 5g daily (no cycling or loading required). On the days you train, throw this in your post-workout shake. On your non-training days, simply have it with breakfast.

2.   **<u>Protei</u>**n – As needed to meet daily protein intake needs, a must for all muscle builders intra and/or post-workout.

3.   Whey concentrate, casein protein, or protein blend - As needed to meet daily protein intake needs, to be reserved for meal replacement needs and pre-bed.

4.   **<u>Carb Powder</u>** – As needed to meet daily carbohydrate needs, to be reserved for intra and post-workout needs only. An absolute must for maximizing performance and recovery.

5.   **<u>Caffeine</u>** – 1-2 caps 30mins prior to training no more than 3-4x per week.

6.   **<u>Citrulline</u>** – 6g of citrulline malate 30mins prior to training, 3.2g beta alanine throughout the day. Beta-alanine can be taken at anytime at your own convenience as it does not have an immediate pre- or post-workout benefit

7.   **<u>Amino Acid Drink (BCAA</u>**)– Take one serving during training if you are not using whey isolate during training.

NOTES: The muscle building protocol is quite self-explanatory; I like to add these nutrients into the big picture meal plan when an athlete is in need of a greater amount of lean muscle mass. Each of these nutrients is demonstrated beneficial and safe within the domain of muscle building, but also provide an energy system specific performance benefit for those who weight train. Although not a "must", this stack has proven time and time again with my clientele to help accelerate muscle building results and get hard-gainers to start putting some size on.

Joint health and joint pain management protocol:

Each of these may be purchased separately or you can utilize the complex from

<u>BioTrust - Joint 33X</u>

1. Glucosamine sulfate – 500mg, 3x daily with food.

2. Chondroitin – 200-400mg, 3x daily with food.

3. **<u>Purathrive Turmeric</u>** - 2x daily with food.

4. **<u>Vitamin C</u>** – 600mg-1g daily with food.

NOTES: Pain during training is in many cases the nature of the beast, I don't think anybody puts a bar on their back, adds a bunch of plates to it and has the idea that they're never going to have pain in their life. It happens to the best of us, but, many people needlessly endure more pain than they need to on a regular basis. The above nutrients and doses are "go-to's" for me to support both the joint structure integrity and the pain management of that structure. Working to both build up joint tissue structure, and keep pain at bay. Although it should be mentioned, often times pain is a result of a poor movement pattern or a structural integrity issue. Make sure technique is spot on, and if you think you have a structural issue it is smart to have a respected authority in your area have a look at it. Oh, and if you're wondering why I included a joint pain protocol in a sleep book, try asking anybody with chronic joint pain how well they're sleeping.

Go ahead, try it.

Trouble falling asleep protocol:

You can buy each of these separately or try this complex from **ATP - Optisom** which contains all of them.

1.   Perform daily ritual within 90mins of bed time

2.   Follow 10-Rules for engineering the perfect night's sleep

3.   **Magnesium**– 200-400mg daily, taken in split doses with your last two meals of the day.

4.   L-Theanine – 200mg taken at 4pm, 200mg taken at 7pm, followed up by a final 200mg taken at 9pm.

5.   Sublingual melatonin – 500mcg 30mins before bed. From here, increase your dose 500mcg per week every week until you find your personal effective dose, or, reach the max dose of 5mg.

NOTES: One of the complaints I get the most often is that people just can't relax and aren't sleeping well. These are the nutrients and doses I use to help sedate people and calm down their body and mind to prepare for a good quality sleep. It is my experience that this stack is strong enough for almost everybody that has ever taken it, and that it dramatically improves somebody's ability to fall asleep. This becomes even more amplified with proper execution of the 10-Rules and the Rituals.

Trouble staying asleep protocol:

You can buy each of these separately or try this complex from **ATP -**

Optisom which contains all of them.

1.   Perform daily ritual within 90mins of bedtime

2.   Follow 10-Rules for engineering the perfect night's sleep

3.   **Magnesium** – 200-400mg daily, taken in split doses with your last two meals of the day.

4.   Sustained release melatonin - 500mcg 30mins before bed. From here, increase your dose 500mcg per week every week until you find your personal effective dose, or, reach the max dose of 5mg

5.   Valerian – 450mg 60mins prior to bedtime

6.   **GABA** – 3-5g taken in the evening, 60mins prior to bedtime

7.   Blood sugar stabilizing nutrient **Biotrust - IC-5 – 1** cap with last meal of the day

NOTES: This protocol is for the population of people that seem to have no problem at all falling asleep, but they wake up several times throughout the night. This can interrupt your sleep wave cycles dramatically and therefore, affect everything we have discussed throughout this information book. Use this protocol to keep the body in a rested state throughout the night so you wake up tomorrow feeling rejuvenated and ready to go.

Trouble falling and staying asleep protocol (also recommended protocol for shift workers):

You can buy each of these separately or try this complex from **ATP - Optisom** which contains all of them.

1.   Perform daily ritual within 90mins of bedtime

2.   Follow 10-Rules for engineering the perfect night's sleep

3.   **Magnesium**– 200-400mg daily, taken in split doses with your last two meals of the day.

4.   Sustained release melatonin – 2mg 30mins prior to bedtime

5.   Sublingual melatonin – 2mg 30mins prior to bedtime

6.   L-Theanine – 200mg taken at 4pm, 200mg taken at 7pm, followed up by a final 200mg taken at 9pm. - Adjust accordingly for earlier or later bedtimes

7.   **GABA** - 3-5g taken in the evening, 60mins prior to bedtime

8.   Lavender – 80-160mg 30-45mins prior to bedtime

NOTES: This is essentially the "Grand Daddy" protocol, the home run. If you have major issues with your sleeping habits, this is the protocol to work into your habits.

Muscle building sleep protocol:

1.   Perform daily ritual within 90mins of bedtime

2.   Follow 10-Rules for engineering the perfect night's sleep

3.   **Magnesium** – 200-400mg daily, taken in split doses with your last two meals of the day.

4.   **Protein Blend or Casein Protein** – 30-40g of protein prior to bedtime

5.   **Glutamine** – 15g of glutamine prior to bedtime, mixed in

your protein shake

6.   Two tbsp. natural peanut butter mixed in your protein shake

7.   **Creatine monohydrate** – 5g in pre-bed shake

8.   Ashwangandha – 300mg at 4pm, 300mg at 7pm

NOTES: The body has a function known as the "Protein Turnover Rate" that is happening inside of us 24hrs a day, 7-Days a week. Within protein turnover, two things are happening simultaneously:

a)   Protein is being added to muscle tissue

b)   Protein is being broken down from muscle tissue

These both operate at different intensities due to various reasons regarding your diet, genetics, training, and time of day. While you're sleeping, it is highly likely that protein breakdown is exceeding protein build up due to the lack of available dietary protein in the bloodstream. We can do two major things to make sure this doesn't happen:

a)   Utilize a slow acting protein powder to supply the body with amino acids during rest so that we can both fight protein breakdown and support protein build up

b)   Utilize a pre-bed dietary fat such as natural peanut butter. Dietary fat dramatically slows the release of food into the bloodstream. Therefore, to our advantage, we can utilize fats pre-bed to ensure a slow stream of amino acids are fed to the muscles during rest to maximally support growth 24hrs a day. Beyond this, fat has been demonstrated several times within the research to have a positive impact on anabolic hormone levels, maximizing the process even further (**Volek, JS. 1997**)

Understanding this, we utilize a protein blend + natural peanut butter as a pre-bed anabolic shake. We combine this with glutamine as it has been shown in some data to support the anabolic response we can get from a meal as well as support our immune system recovery, and we add creatine as well for it's many benefits that it plays towards our strength, power, and lean muscle mass gain.

Lastly, we add in Ashwagandha due to it's ability to improve sleep quality through its anxiety lowering effects, but also add to our muscle building efforts through its repeated ability in the research to improve testosterone and power output levels (**Andrade, C. 2000** + **Wankhede, S. 2015**).

Fat loss sleep protocol:

1.   Perform daily ritual within 90mins of bedtime

2.   Follow 10-Rules for engineering the perfect night's sleep

3.   **Magnesium**– 200-400mg daily, taken in split doses with your last two meals of the day.

4.   L-glutamine – 15g 30mins before your last meal of the day

5.   **Casein Protein or Protein Blend**– 30-40g prior to bedtime

6.   5-HTP – 150-300mg taken in one serving in the evening

7.   EGCG – 400-500mg taken with food in the evening

NOTES: Some people may be surprised at the idea of a pre-bed fat loss stack, thinking something along the lines of "I'm laying in bed, how can I burn fat?". Well, the reality is that you do still burn fat, **all night**.

Why?

You're fasting.

Our objective then is to try and upregulate this fatty acid burning process so you can sleep n' burn. We start off with glutamine, but timed slightly different as some research has

demonstrated that L-glutamine supplemented prior to a meal resulted in a 49% greater energy expenditure after the meal than the group who did not consume any glutamine whatsoever.

Put simply, glutamine supplementation seemed to create a boost in metabolic rate that not supplementing with it but eating the same meal didn't create. For you, more fat burning while in a rested state (**Iwashita, S. 2006**).

The casein is utilized to support the protein turnover rates (see muscle building notes for explanation here) but we have removed the fat intake to lower overall caloric intake to support our dieting efforts.

5-   HTP has been repeatedly seen within the research to reduce cravings, this can be very advantageous for those looking to drop some body fat as it is normally the evenings where the snacks start coming out. With proper supplementation, we can reduce these snack cravings and allow our diet to feel less like, well, a diet. (**Ceci, F. 1989**)

Lastly, EGCG has been repeatedly demonstrated in the research to have amazing health benefits on our body—helping us with everything from cancer prevention to improved blood cholesterol profiles. But, uniquely to EGCG, it has also been demonstrated to improve fatty acid burning and improve blood sugar control. This is important to care about because not only will this aid in overall fat loss, but, the improved blood sugar control will allow you to stay asleep more efficiently as it is normally blood sugar dysregulations that wake people up in the night. (**Venables, MC. 2008**)

Sleeping detox:

1.   Perform daily ritual within 90mins of bedtime

2.   Follow 10-Rules for engineering the perfect night's sleep

3.   **Magnesium–** 200-400mg daily, taken in split doses with your last two meals of the day.

4.   **Glycine** – 3g of glycine 30-60mins prior to sleep

5.   EGCG– 400-50mg taken with food in the evening

NOTES: This is a great stack for those who find themselves in environments that allow for heavy chemical use such as highly populated cities, or if you work in an auto-shop/machine shop, or if you are a painter, etc. The examples could continue, essentially, if you are subject to a daily stream of chemicals that have been known to absorb and cause issues within the human body; then this stack is a good option for you.

You get a lot of bang for your buck here, the core magnesium supplement in every stack is paying it's dividends towards a seemingly endless array of benefits for you as previously

discussed. But, the glycine here is both a very effective detoxifier (a legitimate one by the way, most detoxifying products on the market are worth nothing) and has been demonstrated in research to improve your sleep quality—subjects reporting waking up feeling more refreshed than control subjects who did not take any glycine (**Kentaro, 2006**)

Lastly, we still carry the fat oxidation and health benefits of green tea with us here, but now introducing you the added benefit that EGCG is also an effective detoxifier.

More sleep, better sleep quality, less body toxicity—not a bad deal!

I typically use this stack every single time a client is in a particularly chemical environment. If not, I go more basic and use one of the above protocols.

To wrap this chapter up, although you could never consider a protocol "essential" for the human body, you **can consider sleep essential for the human body**. So, if you're not meeting your daily sleep quality and sleep length needs; incorporating a protocol would be the next logical move for you in order to have your next breakthrough in your muscle building or fat loss efforts.

Afterword

There will be a group of people who just skim through this book and think "Yeah, I knew all that stuff" before tossing it back onto the shelf or into a digital folder never to be seen again, without giving any of the methods a legitimate try or diving into the provided research.

Another group of people will try to find issues and problems with it, and how it has to be adapted to only this situation under whatever context. This will result in this group doing the same old non-productive training and nutrition they always do in their world of paralysis by analysis. You know these guys, they probably corrected your form on social media while never posting a video or picture of their own.

But, there will be a select group of like-minded and positive people, including the many clientele I have already run through the systems and protocols found within this book, that will keep the information nearby so that they can gather all the necessary tools and begin experimenting towards progress.

I'll save you the discovery and break the news to you now. The overwhelming response I hear from my clientele is that it is **NOT** about the protocols, and it is instead about the person you become after you are finally maximizing your sleep. I consistently get e-mail messages on a weekly basis from past clientele telling me:

"What a difference this has made to my daily energy, instead of working on my sleep I was always just grabbing another cup of coffee. I'm down to just one morning cup of coffee a day now!"

"I have finally gotten below 12% body fat! I have been stuck there for long, thank you so much" "I got my testosterone checked after two months on this program and it has gone up 30%!" "I'm down another two notches on my belt and I fit into that old shirt I told you about!"

The e-mails could go on and on, but I'm not here to finish this book off with success stories. I want to articulate very clearly here that it is the **principles** that are important here. Most people will go through their entire health and fitness journey without ever unlocking the power of a good night's sleep, or having any idea how to harness and activate a parasympathetic state. But, it's the exposure to these techniques through the Sequential Shutdown Method that will carryover into your training, performance, recovery, health, and overall life quality.

Where you go from here is all apart of the wonderful journey that is finding our way towards becoming the best versions of ourselves. I can guarantee you this, if you give these methods an honest shot, you will have more clarity about recovery and what it means to properly fuel performance than any other method I know.

Good luck, and let me know how everything works for you.

Until next time.

SLEEP SLIM TEA RECIPE

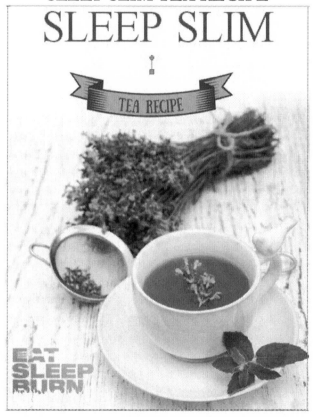

1 SERVING

- 2 tsp Lavender

- 2-3 Tbsp dried Chamomile leaves

- 1 Tbsp of Lemon Balm leaves

- ¼ to ½ tsp Licorice Root

- 2 tsp Ashwagandha powder

- 1 tsp turmeric

- ½ tsp magnesium

- 1/20 of a tsp Magnolia Bark (that is not an error 1/20 is .05 tsp - use small measures to be accurate)

INSTRUCTIONS

Step 1 Bring 8 oz of Milk OR Almond Milk OR Water to a simmer

Step 2 Add Ashwagandha, Turmeric, Magnesium and Magnolia Bark and allow to simmer in pot for 15 minutes. Stir occasionally and do not permit the mixture to boil or burn - keep heat low

Step 3 In kettle Boil 5-8 oz of water

Step 4 Combine Lavender, Chamomile leaves, Lemon Balm, Licorice Root into an infuser or if you don't have one use a fine strainer.

Step 5 Pour boiling water over the leaves into a cup and allow the blend to simmer for 5-7 minutes. Remove the leaf blend from the water

Step 6 Combine milky mixture to the water mixture stir and serve. Allow it to cool to a comfortable temperature

Add a pinch of Cinnamon to taste

If a sweeter taste is preferred - Organic Honey Or Stevia may be used

Lavender

https://www.cupandleaf.com/blog/lavender-tea

Ashwaghanda

https://ascensionkitchen.com/ashwagandha-sleep-tonic/ - **In an exploratory study on healthy volunteers in 2012**, 6 out of 18 participants taking incremental doses of ashwagandha over a 30 day period reported **improvement in quality of sleep**, supporting the traditional use of the herb as a sleep promoter - Study - RAUT, A.A., REGE, N.N., TADVI, F.M., SOLANKI, P.V., KENE, K.R., SHIROLKAR, S.G., ... & VAIDYA, A.B. (2012). EXPLORATORY STUDY TO EVALUATE TOLERABILITY, SAFETY, AND ACTIVITY OF ASHWAGANDHA (WITHANIA SOMNIFERA) IN HEALTHY VOLUNTEERS. Journal of Ayurveda and Integrative Medicine, 3(3), 111-114

- 3-6g daily of the dried root powder / day max

Lemon Balm

https://www.verywellhealth.com/the-health-benefits-of-lemon-balm-89388

Insomnia

The same influence that rosmarinic acid has anxiety is believed to improve sleep in people with insomnia.

According to a 2013 study in Complementary Therapies in Clinical Practice, lemon balm combined with valerian root significantly improve sleep quality in 100 women with menopause when compared to a placebo.

Insomnia and sleep apnea, often accompanied by depression and anxiety, are common features of menopause. The combination of herbs is believed to aid in sleep by acting directly on GABA receptors in the brain, delivering a mild sedative effect while stimulating the production of the "feel-good" hormone serotonin.

Lemon balm may interact with other drugs, including:

Thyroid medications like Synthroid (levothyroxine)

Blood thinners like Coumadin (warfarin) or Plavix (clopidogrel)

Glaucoma medications like Travatan (travoprost)

Chemotherapy drugs like tamoxifen and Camptosar (irinotecan)

In some cases, the drug doses may need to be separated by several hours to avoid interactions. In others, a dose reduction or change of medication may be needed.

Chamomile Leaves

https://www.healthline.com/nutrition/teas-that-help-you-sleep

Stir two to three tablespoons of crushed **chamomile** flowers in a cup of boiling water. Allow the **tea** to steep for five to 10 minutes, then strain and drink.

Magnolia Bark

https://thesleepdoctor.com/2018/02/27/magnolia-bark-affects-sleep-health/

https://selfhacked.com/blog/health-benefits-magnolia-bark/

The recommended dosage for magnolia bark extract is around 250 – 500 mg daily, depending on your desired effects.[2] If you're looking to improve your sleep, a higher dosage of magnolia bark extract is recommended. People use a lower dosage for reducing stress and maintaining good health.

https://www.psychologytoday.com/ca/blog/sleep-newzzz/201809/is-magnolia-bark-the-missing-link-your-sleep-and-health

Licorice Root

https://www.ncbi.nlm.nih.gov/pubmed/22543233

https://selfhacked.com/blog/licorice/

LIMITLESS POTENTIAL SYSTEM

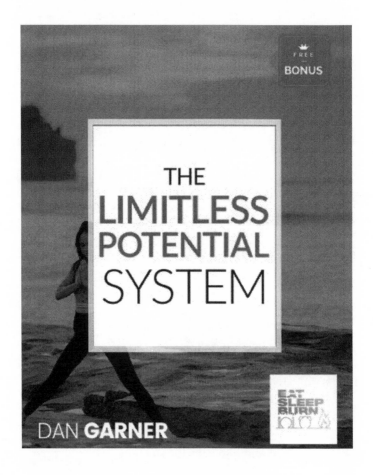

Eat, Sleep, Burn:

The Limitless Potential Guide

Recovery is one of the most important aspects to focus on in the world of physique transformation and maximum performance. Without adequate recovery, subsequent performance is going to suffer as well as progress in the gym will be impossible to gain.

Let that sink in for a second.

If you're not recovered, you will not be taking another step forward in your development in becoming the best version of yourself, and you can even have a high potential in taking a step backwards.

You can think of recovery like a ditch. Every time you train, play a sport, do an intense hobby, have a bad sleep, feel stressed, or go off your diet; you're digging a hole. How big of a hole depends on the intensity of the factor involved. If you strength trained, did conditioning, went on a hike with your friends, and went off the meal plan yesterday, odds are you dug a pretty deep ditch.

Recovery on the other hand is refilling that ditch. When you're on point with your meal planning, sleep quality, sleep length, properly allocated training volume, programed deloads/light weeks, good supplementation, parasympathetic activation, and other advanced recovery strategies you're refilling the ditch so that you're back to where you were.

If you don't refill that ditch every time you dig it, you can't build upon it. Meaning, if you're not fully recovered, you're not going to be making any progress anytime soon. Not only will you not be making progress but you also won't be performing to your potential either due to the effects under recovering has on the body overtime, most commonly known as overtraining syndrome.

So what does that mean for the average gym go'er who does weight training and cardio workouts to look their best, whether it be from a muscle building or fat loss standpoint?

It means you have to be smart about your recovery now, or you will be forced to later.

When you begin to accumulate more fatigue than your body can handle in its current regime a series of issues start to present themselves. Meaning, if you're training very hard with the intent on making serious progress and you're accumulating more fatigue on your body than your current intake of nutrition, sleep quality, sleep length, endocrine, and immune systems can deal with, you will knock over the first domino in the 4-point fatigue line.

FOUR STAGES OF FATIGUE PROGRESSION

#1: Technique

As the onset of fatigue sets in, the first thing to go is technical ability. Remember, lifting weights and cardio conditioning can be extremely technical and demands you move methodically under very high levels of force. All your body parts, distribution of weight and bracing has be working completely in tune while trying to accomplish this. Much easier said than done.

all sorts of things you don't want to run into such as injuries, structural imbalances, cheating with a lot of momentum in lifts, not going through a full range of motion, and just not getting the most bang for your buck out of your workouts. It's not a wild phenomenon that those

Improper technique can lead to guys you see quarter-squatting in the squat rack also have no quads. They have no quads because their technique isn't allowing them to actually train their quads, the only thing that's getting a workout in at that point is their egos.

As a side note away from fatigue progression, I never really understood why people cheat with their lifts. The only person you're cheating is yourself. Using momentum instead of musculature or decreasing the range of motion so you can try and put more weight on the bar and look like a cool guy only ends up decreasing your own progress, muscle mass, fat loss, strength, and performance in the long run while simultaneously increases your risk for injury.

Look, don't be that person. Bad technique creates bad physiques and non-functional bodies. The longer you take to realize that, the longer you will be neglecting your own progress. The ego needs to be left at the door when you enter the gym, progress will come with time and proper execution.

#2: Progress

The second domino that fatigue knocks over is your progress, both in sports (if you compete in anything) and in the gym. You may be able to maintain your current level of strength and physical ability for a period of time. But the actual progression of that strength and level of ability will come to a halt. This is due to a variety of factors including:

•Fatigue decreases overall concentrations of anabolic (muscle building) hormones in the body

•Fatigue increases overall concentrations of catabolic (muscle breakdown) hormones in the body

•Decrease technical skill being the first thing that goes

•Decrease mental capacity for hard training ("I'm just not feeling it today" type of self-talk)

#3: Performance

Third in line to be struck down from the accumulation of fatigue going unchecked is your current level of performance. As mentioned in the previous point your progress will come to a halt and you will be at a standstill, or some would call a "plateau" with your current level of fitness.

But once you have reached this point even your current level of strength and fitness will begin to decline to a lower level. As an extreme example, just think about when you're tired versus when you're not tired.

If somebody asked you to perform a 1RM in the bench press in the middle of the day after you have had a couple of meals versus if somebody woke you up at 3AM to do a 1RM bench press.

Which one do you feel you're going to perform better in? Unless you're a bat or a vampire, you're going to go with option A.

You can think about accumulated fatigue the same way except over a longer period of time. As fatigue gradually increases, performance and results will identically decrease in an inverse relationship.

Always remember that ditch, your job with recovery is to refill that ditch before the next workout. But if you keep digging and digging, you're going to be stuck in a hole of overtraining and your current levels of strength, fitness and performance will all decline.

#4: Injuries

The last and worst thing to happen here that fatigue will eventually cause is an injury. The combination of #1, #2 and #3 is a recipe for disaster and it is only a matter of time before an overworked, under recovered trainee is going to get hurt.

For example, a decrease in technical ability combined with a decrease in performance can create a situation where somebody picks a weight he/she used to be able to do well for eight reps but can only do now for six reps. But he/she is stubborn and wants to be an alpha so he/she breaks technical form a bit during the last two reps so that he/she can squeak out a set of eight but in that technical breakdown in the last two reps a ligament is torn.

Simply put, if you don't make time for recovery now, your body will force you to make time for recovery later with exhaustion and/or injury.

Of course this is relevant to all people, nobody wants to get hurt. But it is especially relevant for the readers of this program because not only could an injury sideline you for 6 months, you may never come back with the same movement mechanics again and this can affect your ultimate potential and how drastic of a change you can make with your body in a given timeframe.

What if you tear your ACL and then squatting never feels the same again?

Or maybe it might feel the same, but you're scared it will happen again and don't have the same confidence you had before when you're looking to add some weight?

See how important recovery can be? Don't overlook it.

It would be the dumbest thing in the world to tear your ACL and be sidelined for 6-8 months because you were too stubborn to deload and you felt like doing an extra rep so you could beat your last set. Forget that stuff, you need to recover.

CATCHING FATIGUE BEFORE IT ARRIVES WITH LEADING, CONCURRENT, AND LAGGING INDICATORS

The problem I see in fatigue management with many people is they simply don't address it at all or have no way in which to measure it. This is something that has to be addressed because if it isn't, you don't know if you need to back off your training a bit, or if you could even **increase** your training volume a bit.

Understanding the above 4-stage fatigue progression model and combining that with these separate indicators will heavily arm you in your battle against fatigue. An ounce of prevention is worth a pound of cure. Catching things before they progress results in a lot less downtime and a lot more progress.

There are three main categories to keeping up with your rate of fatigue and they are leading, concurrent, and lagging indicators. Let's break each one down so you can prepare yourself this year with as much knowledge as possible towards improving your fatigue management:

LEADING INDICATORS

These are parameters which you can use to see if the onset of fatigue is creeping in. They give you a window to see if fatigue is coming to knock on the door soon. Some leading indicators include:

Poor nutrition: A crappy diet is an easy way to not recover and not make progress. But, it doesn't necessarily have an acute effect on fatigue. Meaning, if you generally eat well all the time and have one bad day, odds are your performance and recovery won't actually suffer the next day provided you get back on track. But if your nutrition stays bad, then this will be a leading indicator to the onset of fatigue. You can expect poor performance if you are out of whack nutritionally for several days, just think about what it's like to do conditioning first day back from vacation.

Sleep: Same thing goes for sleep. If you generally sleep well at night and then you have one bad night's sleep. That's not going to kick off enough fatigue to require adjusting training volume or calorie intake. It also probably won't even have a meaningful effect your performance the next day, provided it's just a standard workout. But if this is something that happens several times weekly, you will be running into fatigue issues and you will be running into them real soon. You know now with the information found in this product that sleep is a very large science all by itself and I can't recommend enough times that you need to be sleeping well every night.

Vertical jump test: The vertical jump test has been used as a measure of fatigue for a long time but it should be considered a leading indicator since it is a power and technique sensitive test. Some days people simply just don't jump as well as they normally do but then sleep, eat, and lift heavy ass weights no problem. This is partly because it is a measure of power (not strength, this are not interchangeable terms), but also partly because it is a test that is sensitive to error in my opinion. It can be tough to get baseline numbers and have a measureable track to follow given that:

a)Their jump technique may get better over time which will alter the results

b)Their body composition may get better over time which will alter the results

c)Their strength may get better over time which will alter the results

d)Delayed Onset Muscle Soreness (DOMS) can also present an obvious problem to jump performance irrespective of total fatigue accumulation

All in all, it's quite easily definable but not very accurately measureable. Sure it's a leading indicator, but I'd also take your results with a grain of salt.

CONCURRENT INDICATORS

These are parameters which you can use to see if the fatigue process has already begun and it is time to take a look at your training and nutrition and see what needs to change. Concurrent means the fatigue accumulation process has already begun to sink in and that you should be addressing it.

An example given above on leading indicators was that you could look out the window and see if fatigue was coming to knock on the door. Well, in the concurrent world fatigue is already at the door and asking if it can come in. Concurrent fatigue accumulation indicators include:

Bar speed / Bar weight: This indicator could be summed up as "How does the bar feel?"

Some weeks you're on and some weeks you're not. There are times when there is a weight on the bar that you have lifted no problem before but it feels heavier this week. How heavy it felt and what speed you moved the bar at both play into concurrent fatigue factors. If it feels heavier than before, odds are highly stacked in the favor of you not being fully recovered and have a little hole filling to do in your ditch.

Reps / Capability: This is a very easy and unavoidable parameter to catch. Simply put, are you working to your potential in the gym?

As an easy example, if you did 5 sets of 5 at 250lbs in the squat last week, and this week you could only squeak out sets of 4 reps, this is a problem. Very clear concurrent indicator that you are digging a hole of fatigue. Get out of the ditch!

You're actually weaker than you were previously (remember from the 4-Step fatigue progression model, this look a whole lot like Stage 3 to me) so it's time to re-evaluate your actions and habits.

The way in which this indicator separates itself from bar speed / bar weight category is in that some cases even though the bar feels heavier than normal and moves slower than normal, you still get all your reps. But within this case, you did not reach your potential and fell short of the target.

Grip trength: Grip strength is the last concurrent indicator of fatigue and has been used as a fatigue indicator test for quite some time now by strength and conditioning coaches. You might be asking:

"Why is the vertical jump test a leading indicator and the grip strength a concurrent indicator if they are both physical tests?"

Good question!

The reason for this is physical fitness characteristic decay rates. Different fitness qualities (Power, strength, aerobic endurance, hypertrophy, etc) decay at different rates when you either:

a)   Don't train to maintain them

b)   Don't train at all

c)   Fall too far into fatigue debt

Where the vertical jump separates itself from grip strength is that the jump is mainly a measure of power and power has a faster decay rate than strength, therefore it is a greater leading indicator as opposed to concurrent indicator. Power is going to go before strength in the fatigue continuum.

How the grip strength test works is you are tested on your morning grip strength at certain intervals and if this grip strength begins to consistently drop, fatigue has concurrently set in.

LAGGING INDICATORS

These are parameters which you can use to see if fatigue has already set in and you did not catch it in time. At this point, deloading and/or light days are a necessity until you recover. Ideally, we wouldn't be here at all and you would have already changed things around at this point.

Heart Rate Variability (HRV): HRV has very good data supporting the fact that you are fatigued, but that's exactly it, you're already fatigued. If you were paying close attention to the concurrent and leading indicators of fatigue management you need not HRV because at this point odds are it's too late. This is a deeper zone of fatigue when compared to the concurrent variables.

Now if you're a coach and you are managing a hundred clients at a time and you need reliable data on their fatigue management this can be a great and convenient way to go to track that many people's fatigue status, but I do believe they should go hand-in-hand with the concurrent and leading variables in that you teach your clients what to look for and/or have them fill out a weekly fatigue questionnaire that includes both the concurrent and leading variables so that you can stay on top of it ahead of time.

Actual performance: This is a no-brainer but must be included for completeness of the indicators. Simply put, if you're psychologically unmotivated to go to the gym or to play your sport, or if you're exhausted during/after workouts and you're performance is suffering, you have likely entered a state representative of lagging fatigue.

Brain coherence: Brain coherence can represent many things and can present itself in different ways. But in a nutshell, if you're feeling too mentally drained to go to practice or go to a game, or if you just straight up don't feel like working out at all, this is a fantastic and obvious sign that you are fatigued. Another way this can present itself is in the weight room. You walk up to do deadlifts with a weight you have handled well before but this time your mind is somewhere else when you're trying to set up, you're extending the rest periods and then even during the set your brain is just constantly telling your body to let go and you need to tap into a large amount of willpower to just hang onto the bar.

That's brain coherence not working in your favor. The body is at all times a survival mechanism and the brain doesn't care how much you deadlift today, it just wants to get back to homeostasis. The couch is the land of homeostasis and survival safety.

If you truly understand and have a firm grip on both the 4-point fatigue progression and all of these indicators, there is no reason you should be running into overtraining syndrome. But having said that, in order to make progress we have to place an overload on the body. Meaning, each and every subsequent session you perform must in some way, shape or form be harder than the last.

This is how we place an overload on the body, disrupt homeostasis and force new positive changes to happen and progress to be made (we have to break ourselves down to build ourselves up). The reason I am mentioning this is because you cannot present an overload on the body without causing fatigue. This is of course why easy workouts that don't cause any fatigue also don't give us massive results.

Fatigue can come in the form of:

- Substrate depletion (Phosphocreatine, glycogen)

- Metabolic by-product accumulation (lactate, hydrogen ions)

- Heat + muscle temperature

- Neuromuscular fatigue / neuromuscular transmission (acetylcholine, cholinesterase, electrolyte balance)

- Psychological fatigue

- Impaired sympathetic nervous system

- Impaired parasympathetic nervous system

- Aerobic overtraining

- Anaerobic overtraining

When you're going to the gym 4-6x per week, you're subject to all of the above at some point in your life. Let's make it clear, I am not saying within this manual that you should never be fatigued. That is impossible to happen and you would never make any progress. Fatigue debt is part of the process. We have to dig that ditch in order to rebuild it.

With the above indicators and progressions I was simply arming you with the awareness to avoid too much fatigue. Some fatigue is ok, too much is a bad thing which causes several problems as mentioned earlier.

Now that you know what to look for, let's discuss some strategies which you can use with your training for optimal recovery between physical bouts.

EAT, SLEEP, BURN: RECOVERY STRATEGIES

Recovery being one of the most important aspects towards progress and performance in any physical endeavor, you think that it would require the same amount of respect and attention to detail as coaches give the other components of fat loss, muscle building and performance such as technique, nutrition, strength training, conditioning, and mobility. Unfortunately it's just not the case.

From my observation, many coach's kind of just lump all recovery strategies into one "Post-Workout Recovery" category and let that be that. They use the same recovery strategies for almost every scenario and feel that that's an adequate response. This is a big error to make, not only because different states of overtraining have different implications on the body, but also because different recovery strategies have their own cost/benefit analysis to them. If we throw the kitchen sink of recovery at every athlete there is a high chance we are doing them a disservice. To recover smarter, it's important to understand the what affects what and how this presents itself in the picture of overall performance.

For example, volume related overtraining has been shown to increase cortisol and decrease resting luteinizing hormone and total/free testosterone concentrations. However, intensity related overtraining does not appear to alter resting concentrations of testosterone, free testosterone, cortisol or growth hormone. Apples and oranges here. This is just one of the many examples where recovery strategies used differentiate themselves from one another.

Instead of diving into the seemingly endless research on the topic, let's make things simple and categorize them:

1. General recovery strategies

2. Exercise related recovery strategies

3. Short term vs. Long term recovery

GENERAL RECOVERY STRATEGIES

General recovery for the purpose of this discussion is going to be defined as certain recovery strategies in which provide so many benefits towards multiple systems in the body that they are not specific to any one category. Additionally, it is the general recovery strategies that are the most important to focus on before moving into more advanced categories. General recovery includes attention to:

1.Sleep

2.Calories

SLEEP

Sleep gets the number one slot here because sleep is the king of fatigue management, even people who don't train or play sports can tell you that. No matter how many massages, Epsom salt baths, supplements, food or anything you do cannot make up for a bad night's sleep. No matter what, you're going to be tired and you're not going to have fully recovered from your previous training session. There's no way around that and no, taking more caffeine doesn't override it either. Caffeine isn't a bad thing, but if you need large amounts of it to function every day you could probably do with some sleep quality enhancement.

Sleep is especially important because while you're sleeping, nearly all systems are anabolic. Bones, muscles and the endocrine system are all synthesizing materials and adapting to the overload you placed on it.

Muscles are of course creating new contractile proteins, bones adding calcium/phosphorus, and the endocrine system is increasing levels of testosterone, IGF-1, growth hormone and thyroid hormones. All extremely important factors to progress in the gym and with your health. Not to mention sleep is also a regulator of your respiratory exchange ratio, which determines how much of your metabolic rate you are burning at rest is coming from either lean muscle tissue or fatty tissue. This is very important to care about because regardless of your dietary strategy or how you train, the quality of your sleep can still decrease lean muscle tissue within the body.

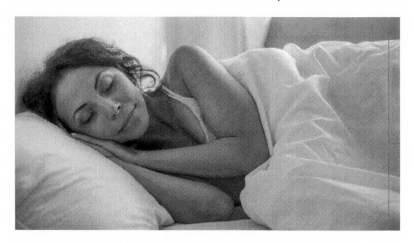

Strategies to improve the quality of your sleep include:

• Adequate hydration throughout the day

• Completely pitch black room to sleep in

• Unplug all electrical equipment in your room

• Do not have your phone on or use it as an alarm

• Getting up and going to bed at the same time every day and night

• Using different strategies to bring stress down throughout the day

• Writing down what you need to accomplish tomorrow or what you don't want to forget so that it may leave your mind and you can relax pre-bed.

• Try to calm down at night time. Nobody ever went to bed relaxed and ready to properly sleep just after watching UFC or action movies. Not going to happen. Reading leisurely (not researching or planning) is a great way to calm down and prime your body for rest.

• No TV within 2hrs of bedtime

• Not having every light on in the house after 6pm. The body responds to light as if it is day time and this can delay the proper production of melatonin, a sleep hormone that is necessary for you to be able to fall asleep and stay asleep

One last thing that is important to note, is there is no optimal amount of sleep, there is only an optimal amount of sleep for you. Some people only need 7hrs, some people need up to 10hrs per night. The idea is to get enough to where you feel best. If you can function throughout the day at a high level without massive doses of caffeine, then you're probably good. But if you are chronically under rested, it should be your #1 priority before moving on to anything else.

A good rule I like to use is that you should never wake up with an alarm. This gets people out of the idea of thinking they have to sleep 8 or 9hrs. If 7hrs is good for you and you're not being interrupted by an alarm doing this, by all means go for it. It should also be noted here that "more is better" isn't true. You will not be gaining any advantage sleeping 14hrs a night if your body doesn't need to for adequate recovery. Simply waking up without an alarm is ensuring you are doing it right and that your body is determining when it is ready for the day.

CALORIES

I say calories because calories in and of themselves are more important than the macronutrients they are being derived from (protein, carbs, fat). The total greater energy load you are getting in is more important than where they are coming from, provided you aren't completely screwing it up and running a dumb meal plan that makes no sense for performance. I'm cutting you some slack here and assuming you aren't eating candy and fast food every day.

Although with calories, the "more is better" strategy is actually true but only up to a point. You want to be taking in as many calories as possible but it's no excuse to start gaining body fat, that's completely counterproductive to both muscle building and fat loss optimization.

To put it short, calories need to be #1 on your nutritional priorities list for recovery. This includes fat loss, muscle building and optimal performance. You can't escape it, it is your most powerful tool for permanent body composition change and without it the other nutritional strategies effectiveness becomes much less pronounced if even existent at all.

Calories need to be there for fatigue management because you need to not only eat back what you lost during training, but also eat enough in order to give your body the raw materials to construct new muscle mass with. Muscle and recovery cannot be created through thin air, it needs calories. The way in which you control them ultimately determines how successful you are with your nutrition.

I can't stress enough the importance of these two general recovery strategies. They affect all systems within the body, how well you focus on them determines if that effect is either positive or negative.

There is no real sense in moving forward to other strategies until these two are nailed down. For example, if you're sleeping 4 hrs a night and you go out to get a massage to improve recovery, nothing is going to happen. That level of sleep is going to prevent you from recovering no matter what.

In another example, if you're under eating 500 calories a day and your goal is to put on muscle mass so you take a recovery supplement throughout the day to boost recovery. It doesn't matter how awesome or how expensive that recovery supplement is, at the end of the day you're under eating so you're not recovering and you're definitely not going to gain any weight.

These two have to be in check regardless of the goal at hand. Once these two are nailed down and you feel recovery could still use a boost, then you may move forward into the more advanced and specific strategies.

EXERCISE RELATED RECOVERY STRATEGIES

Exercise related recovery strategies are just that, recovery modalities with the intent on refilling the ditch that exercise built and not necessarily other components within one's life (sleep, stress, etc). The primary mechanism for fatigue from exercise is substrate depletion.

For you, this means the depletion of carbohydrates and phosphocreatine energy stores from within the body. Let's talk about some of the problems and best practical strategies you can use in your programming today to start recovering better from all of your weight training and cardio sessions.

PCR DEPLETION

Phosphocreatine (PCr) is first in line for energy substrate use in anaerobic conditions. What does that mean for you? It is first in line for energy substrate use both during your intense cardio work and in the gym. PCr intramuscular storage plays a critical role in performance and although

we create our own natural creatine every day (Approx. 1g), it is wise to supplement as well to maximize the amount of available creatine you have to delay fatigue and increase force output. The majority of all weight training sets happen in less than 20 secs and place a heavy emphasis on a high rate of force production, from a physiological perspective this cannot be overlooked and should be a focus for refilling your ditch.

Strategies to help offset this fatigue are simple:

•   Supplement with 5-10g creatine monohydrate daily for maximum availability and intramuscular storage

•   Ensure there is no pre-mature exhaustion of PCr prior to strength training or cardio. Meaning, no high power work sessions or excessive warm ups prior to important workouts

•   Improvements in alactic conditioning

GLYCOGEN DEPLETION

Glycogen is the stored form of energy within the muscle and liver cells coming from carbohydrates in the diet. Carbohydrates are the most important energy substrates to be around in anybody's diet who is looking for maximum body composition change in the shortest possible timeframe. This is especially true before, during and after workouts.

Although PCr turns on first, it does not last very long. An adequate glycogen / glucose flow in the body can keep you performing optimally the entire duration of the workout, but when levels are low, performance dramatically suffers. We have known this in the scientific literature for a long time, carbohydrates improve performance under all sorts of conditions. We need to drive performance to its highest levels and carbohydrates are both the preferred fuel source for the muscular system and the nervous system. Delaying both local and systemic fatigue during your training sessions.

Strategies to offset this major contributor to fatigue on the field include:

- Proper meal plan design for your goals

- Pre/during/post workout liquid nutrients

METABOLIC BY-PRODUCTS

Lactic acid is a by-product of anaerobic work and although most people believe that lactic acid is responsible for fatigue in all type of exercise, lactic acid accumulates within the muscle fiber only during relatively brief, highly intense muscular effort. Take for example marathon runners, they have near resting levels of lactic acid levels at the end of a race, despite their fatigue. Their fatigue is much more as a result of inadequate energy supply as opposed to a rise in blood lactate.

Weight training on the other hand, is susceptible to lactic acid accumulation (then converting to lactate), as well as the production of hydrogen ions; the combination of which giving the "burning" sensation during competition. The body can only buffer this acidifying effect for so long before a threshold is hit and fatigue shuts down muscular contraction. You can compare this feeling to when the muscles are burning to a point where you are forced to stop.

Strategies to delay the inevitable here include:

- Supplementation with creatine monohydrate and beta-alanine which have both been shown to act as a buffer and delay the onset on lactate/hydrogen ion accumulation

• Improvements in conditioning levels improve the rate at which you can delay this fatiguing process

• Keeping an optimal electrolyte balance within the body is crucial for recovery and the recycling of this lactate back into the energy system

OFF DAYS

Simply a day off from the gym! If you wake up exhausted, mentally drained and have no desire to go to the gym, staying home is probably a better idea than going in. This is known in the scientific world as passive recovery.

It's very important to separate this from laziness. Passive recovery is required not often, but when it is it can be a smart thing to do. Simply stay home, partake in an activity that makes you happy, destress and decompress. You'll come back stronger tomorrow because of it.

INTENTIONALLY LIGHT SESSIONS

These days are reserved for the days where you think you are ok until you get your first couple of sets or runs in. If they feel terrible, heavier than normal and feel like a chore, this might be a good day to have a light day.

You're already at the gym or out on the field so let's get something in but drop it down to your current level so that we don't dig a deeper ditch of recovery debt here. An important guideline to follow is that I don't want you to drop intensity (weight on the bar), I want you to drop 50% of your volume. Meaning, if you normally squat 300lbs for

4 x 10. You would still use 300lbs, but instead do 2 x 10. This is best case scenario to ensure you don't back track at all but still allow recovery processes to occur.

SEQUENCE OF LIGHT SESSIONS (DELOAD)

Research has shown that performing light sessions can actually be more beneficial towards recovery than doing nothing. On top of this, light sessions are much better towards preventing any fitness decay rates from occurring (the loss of strength, muscle or power). A deload should be in place within your training periodization every 4-6 weeks depending on the intensity and volume of the training program.

This recovery period will allow you to fully adapt from the training stimuli while simultaneously fully recovering you to go all out for another training program. This is known within the scientific world as active recovery.

ACTIVE REST PHASE: 1-3 WEEKS

Active rest normally follows brutal competition and a long time of being beat up and working hard. For you, this normally means taking a couple weeks off of any intense physical activity you partake in and your training once per year, usually right after the most grueling stretch. If you play hockey for example, you would incorporate this right after the season.

Once per year it's wise for anybody to take at least a couple weeks off to allow some nagging injuries to heal and to get his/her hunger for competition and training back. It is not advised to do nothing during this phase though, just stay out of the gym and off whichever other physical activities you are involved in. Active rest phases should typically incorporate low intensity, fun activities such as:

- Hiking

- Recreation basketball

- Walking around the park everyday

- Recreation tennis

- Swimming

HEAT + MUSCLE TEMPERATURE

Exercise in excessive heat increases carbohydrate utilization and can speed up glycogen depletion. It has been hypothesized throughout sports science that increased muscle temperatures impair both muscle function and muscle metabolism. Exercising in temperatures of 11 – 21 degrees Celsius show greatest performance benefits while exercising below 4, or above 31 creates the quickest times to fatigue.

Strategies to offset this are straight forward, train in a suitable environment and dress accordingly. Training in the boiling hot weather or freezing cold does not "toughen you up". It's a poor strategy for improving performance and detracts from the rate of progress you could be making otherwise.

MANUAL THERAPY

Practices such as chiropractic, massage, fascial stretch therapy, and active release therapy can play a meaningful role in one's recovery from sports and exercise. Each of these practices (and many more I probably forgot to mention) have proven benefits to them on increasing the rate of recovery among many other things health related in which each practice brings different benefits and is suitable for different situations.

Having said this, this is of course beneficial towards recovery but only up to a certain point. Extremes have been seen in this world where 300lbs Helga digs her thumbs into your muscles and tears you apart. Trauma is trauma, it's as simple as that. There's a reason that it hurts for a few days after the massage just like a workout would. This in most cases can be good for something, but not acute recovery from exercise. Any stress beyond a point placed on the body post-workout can be a detriment to the recovery adaptation process that is supposed to be taking place.

In the discussion of recovery alone, if you're out getting massages but your sleep and diet are off, you're not doing yourself any favors. You would be much better off putting that money towards correcting your sleep and hopping on a good meal plan made by a specialist. Those two will take you a long ways before you will ever need manual therapy work; that is unless you have issues outside of basic muscle and nervous system recovery that require manual therapy such as structural, skeletal and/or fascial issues.

SHORT TERM VS. LONG TERM RECOVERY

As mentioned towards the beginning of this manual, I feel coaches far too often clump recovery strategies all into the same category. Having read this far into it you are now much more knowledgeable about this topic and can not only track and measure your rate of fatigue, but also hand pick some of the best strategies in order to optimally recover from both sport and exercise.

That's a powerful thought right there.

Understanding how important recovery is can be a big "aha!" moment for you all by itself. Now you can not only discuss the ins and outs of recovery but also apply those strategies as well. Talking the talk is cool and all so you can look smart at a dinner party, but without application it doesn't mean a whole lot.

Which brings us to our last category for optimal recovery, which isn't so much of a statement as it is a question:

"Do you need to perform at your best now? Or can you perform later?"

In other words, do you need super accelerated recovery strategies for short term recovery so that you can perform at your best again very soon, or can you use more standard recovery strategies because performance isn't a priority right now?

Most will undoubtedly say "Well, short term! Let's perform now man, why would I wait?"

Because recovery strategies, like everything else in the strength and conditioning world, also have a cost/benefit analysis to them. It is this category which is one of the biggest reasons why I even categorize recovery modalities.

Let's use a credit card analogy so that I can paint a picture for you and describe why you have to separate short term vs. long term.

Credit card balance is at $0.00

I want you to imagine that $0.00 is your current level of fitness right now. As it stands, that figure is representative of how fit you are and how well you perform in present day.

Now, let's say you worked out very hard today, 10 sets of 10 on the barbell squat plus a bunch of other lower body work. That's going to trash your legs and you better bet that's going to create a fatigue debt.

Now you're at -$20.00 on your fatigue credit card. Just like the ditch was dug earlier, this is a different representation of that fatigue debt.

So now you're in debt. You can pay off that debt the long term way and put $5.00 on it every day for the next 4 days. But when you pay it off this long term way, the bank gives you a bonus and adds $5.00 to your account.

So as it stands right now, the fatigue debt from the leg workout brought you back to -$20.00 on your credit card but through long term money management and a bank bonus you were able to get back +$5.00 in your account.

Remember I said earlier that your base level of fitness was $0.00?

Well now it's at $5.00. You have now made progress and are a better, stronger person for it.

That's long term recovery strategy played out in numbers.

But there's a short term way as well. You met a dude in a dark alley who can cheat and slash your credit card from -$20.00 right back to $0.00 over night. But you don't want to tell the bank and receive the $5.00 reward just in case you get caught and get in trouble.

So where does short term extreme methods of recovery leave you?

Well, you went from -$20.00 back to $0.00. So you recovered from that given session, but you didn't actually make any progress.

That right there is one of the most important things you will read within this manual.

Short term extreme recovery modalities such as contrast showers, ice baths, cryotherapy, etc, all have their place during a certain time of the year as they can create rapid recovery and have you ready to go the next day. But at the same time, they decrease adaptations gained from the gym.

Meaning, if you and your buddy both hit a hard leg workout today and you took an ice bath afterwards and he didn't, he will have made the better progress from the workout. You may have recovered quicker, but he will ultimately have gained more progress from the session.

That's important to care about because it opens our eyes to a couple different scenarios.

#1: It would not be very smart to try and use all these short term advanced recovery strategies if you're trying to build muscle and strength. With these goals, short term strategies actually end up hurting your progress.

#2: It would be very smart to utilize these strategies during times at which you are expected to perform at the best of your ability day in and day out, without muscle/strength gain being the top priority. Such as during a competitive season of baseball. The competitive sports seasons, especially in certain weeks where you have to play several times in the same week (playoffs) demand your best performance everyday.

The in-season is not about bringing your muscle and strength up, it's about performing. If you're under recovered and you're expected to perform on the field tomorrow, an ice bath or contrast shower can be a great idea.

Why?

Because progress in the gym isn't the #1 priority right now, performance on the field is.

If you don't understand the difference between short term and long term recovery I want you to re-read that whole section before moving on to reading about the advanced short term recovery strategies. It's very important you understand both the positives and the negatives towards using extreme recovery strategies.

For practicality reasons, I will not be discussing Normatec or cryotherapy as most people do not have access to these at home or on the road. I will only be discussing two of the most popular and most practical strategies, contrast showers and ice baths.

CONTRAST SHOWERS

The contrast shower approach offers many of the same supposed benefits that ice baths do, just without the ice. It is a slightly more comfortable approach (not sure if comfortable is still the right word though!) then the ice baths and still may boost recovery rate so you can get in the gym faster and train harder.

Give them a shot if you feel they work for you, there is an army of people who use them. In the research, it is quite inconclusive. If you find this works for you, I like it as this is something you can do at home or at any hotel or vacation.

The protocol for contrast showering varies between which coaches you talk to. The method I use requires a shower, and a stop watch. Keep things practical so that when you're on the road it's still doable.

It's important to keep a timing device around because you are going to be spending more time in the heat then you are the cold, and going by time keeps you honest, if you go by feel you will cheat yourself out of the uncomforting temperatures that will be providing benefit.

You begin with hot water, and switch to cold water. Then, through each cycle, you make the hot hotter, and the cold colder. By the last round it should be uncomfortably hot and uncomfortably cold. It is also important to note that you always want to end on cold. After the shower, quickly warm up with a towel.

The durations of these can vary based on how much time you have and also how grueling the workout was. The back to back hot / cold environment creates a "pump" effect in the muscles which can improve the removal of exercise produced waste products. Which are the main things that drive soreness and inflammation in your muscles in the days after training. Here's how it breaks down:

STANDARD PROTOCOL

- 3-4 cycles

- 3 minutes of hot

- 1 minute of cold

- Finish on cold

LIGHT PROTOCOL

- 2-3 cycles

- 1 minute hot

- 30 secs cold

- Finish on cold

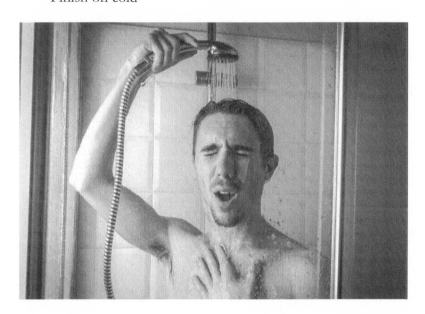

ICE BATHS

The consensus on this style of recovery strategy is that the exposure to cold helps to combat the micro-trauma and acute inflammation within the muscle post-exercise and subsequent soreness caused by intense or repetitive activities such as strength training and cardio.

The ice bath acts to constrict blood vessels, flush waste products and reduce swelling and tissue breakdown. Subsequently, as the tissue warms back up after the ice bath the increased blood flow speeds circulation within the targeted area, kick starting that healing process.

The advantage of an ice bath submersion is that a large area of musculature can be treated. Simply hop right in and you've got a total body recovery process started.

Here are some guidelines to follow as you will get many conflicting opinions from different coaches should you ask around:

• Always be conservative with the temperature you choose. Like everything else in life you should start easy and work your way up. Most specialists recommend anywhere from 54-60 degrees Fahrenheit. Start a little higher than here and work your way down if necessary. There's no "look how hardcore I am" award for cold ice baths

• Don't push yourself to do exactly what your teammate or training partner is doing. Everybody has their own thresholds, stay within yours. Again, no cool points for going the longest or the coldest. That's dumb, don't be dumb

• Typical exposure time should be 6-8 mins

• Colder and longer is not better. This is a case where "more is better" does not apply and could become detrimental

• Do not submerge in a warm water or warm shower immediately after the ice bath. Warm yourself gradually with clothes, blankets, towels and a warm meal

As a final topic, I want to briefly discuss protein and carbohydrates and their order of importance in reference to short term vs. long term recovery.

On a long term macronutrient importance scale for recovery, it would run like this:

Protein → Carbohydrates → Fat

But on a short term importance scale such as the example if you're working out twice in one day, or plan on doing a workout and a sports event in the same day, recovery from a macronutrient importance scale looks more like this:

Carbohydrates →Protein → Fat

It doesn't so much matter over a long term period, such as 24hrs because glycogen replenishment is going to occur anyways over that time period. Meaning, if you work out or have a game today, and you don't have any physical activity again on this same day then it's no big deal. Your energy will be back and good to go tomorrow provided you stayed true to your macronutrient and calorie recommendations.

But in a short period between physical activities, such as 4-8 hrs, speed of glycogen replenishment is key to performing at 100% if you're working out again or doing two workouts in the same day. Proper timing strategies must be in place in these scenarios for continual peak performance. This is why carbohydrates come first because carbohydrate timing on these days are crucial.

WHAT ARE THE TAKEAWAYS?

1.   As you progressively accumulate fatigue, at first technique will breakdown both in and out of the gym. Then your progress in strength and conditioning will come to a halt, only to be followed up by an actual decrease in performance. Lastly, what we all don't want, if you let fatigue accumulate enough the combination of all the above will result in injury. Fatigue progression model:

Technique   Progress   Performance   Injury

2.   You must understand that fatigue has many leading, concurrent and lagging indicators. Understanding these in combination with the fatigue progression model gives you a bulletproof checklist for fatigue progression that will allow you to never run into any overtraining issues.

3.   The general recovery strategies are infinitely more important than any of the other recovery strategies. Meaning, if you aren't eating correctly or sleeping well, you need to focus on those first before moving into the more specific recovery strategies.

4.   Once the general recovery strategies have been mastered and you are still running into recovery issues, you can then move on to the more specific interventions such as PcR depletion, glycogen depletion, manual therapy, metabolic by-products, muscle temperature or the need for some time off/light days.

5.   Short term recovery is very different than long term recovery from a physiological standpoint and must be treated as such. Ice baths and contrast showers have their place, but you must always consider performance vs. adaptations.

28 DAY METABOLIC RESET

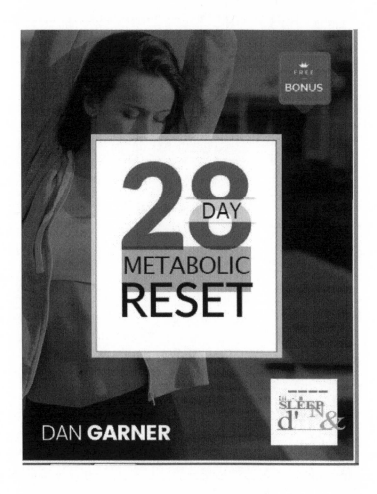

28- Day Metabolic Reset

Make no mistake about it - bodyweight training has been an incredibly effective tool for physique transformation, power development, increasing strength, burning body fat, building muscle tissue, and pushing the limits of human performance for centuries.

Don't believe me?

Convicts, martial artists, gymnasts, developing country athletes, world-famous at-home DVD workout success stories, among many other disciplines will all prove you otherwise. Bodyweight training when done correctly is the real deal.

Bodyweight training is just like any other form of training, overtime you will continue to make linear progress so long as you continue to apply an overload stimulus to each and every workout.

The principal of overload represents your continuous ability to provide the muscle with a stimulus that it has not been exposed to before. Thus, forcing it to adapt and become a better version of itself. How it adapts depends on which type of stimulus you provide it through your training. Your muscle could increase in aerobic conditioning, anaerobic conditioning, strength, power, size, speed, co-ordination, etc…

Overload to a muscle can be provided through an increase in weight you use, an increase in the range of motion you move through, a different angle of movement, a decreased or increased rest period, longer time under tension, isometrics, and any other variation you can think of.

Bodyweight training's only limit is your mind. When you utilized the training principles that we know are deeply rooted within the scientific literature you can design a kick ass bodyweight plan to get you transforming results in a short period of time.

Enter the 28-Day Metabolic Reset.

The 28-Day Metabolic Reset uses the principal of overload to keep things simple, rational, and brutal. Don't get it twisted here either, just because something is bodyweight it doesn't make it easy.

This program isn't for everybody, it's for the people who have the internal drive to push them through and pass the finish line on some seriously great workouts. You follow this plan for the next 28-Days and I promise you two things:

1.   Your body is going to transform

2.   You will understand work ethic and the power of bodyweight training better than anybody you know.

How it works...

For the next 28-Days, you're going to be utilizing multiple techniques and strategies to apply overload on the body to accomplish several physiologic changes simultaneously. Your week is going to be split up into 4 intense workout sessions, each utilizing different metabolic pathways so you can get the greatest response in the shortest possible time. Here's how the schedule looks:

Day 1 – Upper Body Strength and Hypertrophy

Day 2 – Metabolic Conditioning 1

Day 3 – Off

Day 4 – Lower Body Strength and Hypertrophy

Day 5 – Metabolic Conditioning 2

Day 6 – Off

Day 7 – Off

Days 1 and 4 we will be focusing on giving you the foundation of strength and muscle you need so that when you shred the fat off, you have more tone and shape to your physique. These are important to keep in the schedule because those who dismiss this all together tend to still drop body fat, but don't have the lines of definition that they were hoping for once they got lean.

It's kind of like this, the definition you get on your body is like the paint on a house. If you have no house, all you have is a bucket of paint!

We all know somebody whom we would call lean, but they still don't have much definition or an impressive physique. All paint, no house.

The house provides you the foundation you need in order to have an athletic build so that when it's time for the painters to come in, you look your best and create that "whoa" effect on social media with the new picture you just posted.

Beyond this, days 2 and 5 are created with one goal in mind; **to create the maximum amount of fat loss in the shortest possible time without any equipment**. When it starts hurtin', keep it going. Conditioning workouts remind me of a saying my old Tae Kwon Do coach used to say:

"A workout is going to be as hard as you want it to be"

Sure, you could slack off during your intervals and you would still have completed the workout. But, it's not a question of whether you did the workout today, it's a question of how you did it. You want to change your body in 28-Days? You better bring it. Let's go.

28 - Day Metabolic Reset Workout System

WEEK 1

UPPER BODY STRENGTH AND HYPERTROPHY

A1:   Standard push ups 3 x 15

A2:   Inverted row 3 x 15

   Complete both exercises back to back with only 60 secs between rounds

B1:   Supinated chin ups 3 x 8

B2:   Angled bodyweight triceps extension 3 x 15

   Complete both exercises back to back with only 60 secs between rounds

C1:   Downward dog push ups 3 x 10

C2:   Plank 3 x 30 secs

   Complete both exercises back to back with only 60 secs between rounds

METABOLIC CONDITIONING 1

Descending Burpees

Set 1: 20 reps

Set 2: 19 reps

Set 3: 18 reps

Set 4: 17reps

Set 5: 16 reps Etc…

Perform until you get down to 1 rep with a maximum of 30secs rest between sets

LOWER BODY STRENGTH AND HYPERTROPHY

A1:   Hand supported ¼ pistol squats 3 x 8/leg

A2:   Lying single leg hip thrusts 3 x 12/leg

Complete both exercises back to back with only 60 secs between rounds

B1:   Front foot elevated split squat 3 x 8/leg

B2:   Standing calf raises 3 x 25

Complete both exercises back to back with only 60 secs between rounds

C1:   Walking lunges 3 x 10/leg

C2:   Side plank 3 x 15 secs/side

Complete both exercises back to back with only 60 secs between rounds

METABOLIC CONDITIONING 2

A1:   Jump rope for 3 mins

A2:   Speed squats x 25

 A3:   Jump rope for 3 mins

A4:   Bicycle crunches x 15 each side

A5:   Jump rope for 3 mins

A6:   Wide   push   ups   x   15
Complete all six exercises back to back with minimal rest in between
each exercise, and 2 mins rest once completed the sixth exercise.
Repeat for 3 total rounds.

WEEK 2

UPPER BODY STRENGTH AND HYPERTROPHY

A1:   Diamond push ups 3 x 15

A2:   Inverted row with 1sec pause at the top 3 x 15

Complete both exercises back to back with only 60 secs between
rounds

B1:   Supinated chin ups with 1sec pause in the stretched position
3 x 8

B2:   Angled bodyweight triceps extension (walk out a little further
this week) 3 x 15

Complete both exercises back to back with only 60 secs between
rounds

C1: Elevate feet on small box push ups (keep head between shoulders and drive head forward to the ground) 3 x 10

C2: Plank 3 x 35 secs

Complete both exercises back to back with only 60 secs between rounds

METABOLIC CONDITIONING 1

Descending Mountain Climber Burpees

Set 1: 20 reps

Set 2: 19 reps

Set 3: 18 reps

Set 4: 17reps

Set 5: 16 reps Etc…

Perform until you get down to 1 rep with a maximum of 30 secs rest between sets

LOWER BODY STRENGTH AND HYPERTROPHY

A1: Hand supported ½ pistol squats 3 x 8/leg

A2: Lying single leg hip thrusts 3 x 12/leg

Complete both exercises back to back with only 60 secs between rounds

B1: Flat split squat 3 x 8/leg

B2: Standing calf raises with toes elevated 3 x 25

Complete both exercises back to back with only 60 secs between rounds

C1:   Walking lunges 3 x 12/leg

C2:   Side plank 3 x 20 secs/side

Complete both exercises back to back with only 60 secs between rounds

METABOLIC CONDITIONING 2

A1:   Jump rope for 3 mins

A2:   Speed squats x 25

A3:   Jump rope for 3 mins

A4:   Bicycle crunches x 15 each side

A5:   Jump rope for 3 mins

A6:   Wide push ups x 15

Complete all six exercises back to back with minimal rest in between each exercise, and 2 mins rest once completed the sixth exercise. Repeat for 4 total rounds.

WEEK 3

UPPER BODY STRENGTH AND HYPERTROPHY

A1:   Knuckle push ups 3 x 15

A2:   Inverted row with 2 sec pause at the top 3 x 15

Complete both exercises back to back with only 60 secs between rounds

B1:   Supinated chin ups with 2 sec pause in the stretched position 3 x 8

B2:   Angled bodyweight triceps extension (walk out a little further this week) 3 x 20

Complete both exercises back to back with only 60 secs between rounds

C1:   Elevate feet on medium size box push ups (keep head between shoulders and drive head forward to the ground) 3 x 10

C2:   Plank 3 x 40 secs

Complete both exercises back to back with only 60 secs between rounds

METABOLIC CONDITIONING 1

Descending Candlestick Burpees

Set 1: 20 reps

Set 2: 19 reps

Set 3: 18 reps

Set 4: 17reps

Set 5: 16 reps Etc…

Perform until you get down to 1 rep with a maximum of 30 secs rest between sets

LOWER BODY STRENGTH AND HYPERTROPHY

A1:Hand supported ¾ pistol squats 3 x 8/leg

A2:Lying single leg hip thrusts 3 x 12/leg

Complete both exercises back to back with only 60 secs between rounds

B1:Bulgarian split squats 3 x 8/leg

B2:Single leg standing calf raises with toes elevated 3 x 25 per leg

Complete both exercises back to back with only 60 secs between rounds

C1:Walking lunges 3 x 15/leg

C2:Side plank 3 x 25 secs/side

Complete both exercises back to back with only 60 secs between rounds

METABOLIC CONDITIONING 2

A1:Jump rope for 3 mins

 A2:Speed squats x 25

A3:Jump rope for 3 mins

A4:Bicycle crunches x 15 each side

A5:Jump rope for 3 mins

A6:Wide push ups x 15

Complete all six exercises back to back with minimal rest in between each exercise, and 2 mins rest once completed the sixth exercise.

Repeat for 5 total rounds.

WEEK 4

UPPER BODY STRENGTH AND HYPERTROPHY

A1:Hindu push ups 3 x 15

A2:Inverted row with 3 sec pause at the top 3 x 15

Complete both exercises back to back with only 60 secs between rounds

B1:Supinated chin ups with 3 sec pause in the stretched position 3 x 8

B2:Angled bodyweight triceps extension (walk out a little further this week) 3 x 25

Complete both exercises back to back with only 60 secs between rounds

C1:Handstand push up 3 x MAX (go until you are 1-Rep shy of failure)

C2:Plank 3 x 45 secs

Complete both exercises back to back with only 60 secs between rounds

METABOLIC CONDITIONING 1

Descending Tuck Jump Burpees

Set 1: 20 reps

Set 2: 19 reps

Set 3: 18 reps

Set 4: 17reps

Set 5: 16 reps Etc…

Perform until you get down to 1 rep with a maximum of 30 secs rest between sets

LOWER BODY STRENGTH AND HYPERTROPHY

A1:Hand supported full pistol squats 3 x 8/leg

A2:Lying single leg hip thrusts 3 x 15/leg

Complete both exercises back to back with only 60 secs between rounds

B1:Jumping alternating split squats 3 x 8/leg

B2:   Single leg standing calf raises with toes elevated and 1 sec pause in the stretch position 3 x 15 per leg

Complete both exercises back to back with only 60 secs between rounds

C1:Walking lunges 3 x 20/leg

C2:Side plank 3 x 30 secs/side

Complete both exercises back to back with only 60 secs between rounds

METABOLIC CONDITIONING 2

A1:Jump rope for 3 mins

A2:Speed squats x 25

A3:Jump rope for 3 mins

A4:Bicycle crunches x 15 each side

A5:Jump rope for 3 mins

A6:Wide push ups x 15

Complete all six exercises back to back with minimal rest in between each exercise, and 2 mins rest once completed the sixth exercise. Repeat for 6 total rounds.

Made in the USA
Middletown, DE
12 January 2020